P9-BAV-935

Praise for
Thinking Differently

"In pursuit of ensuring an excellent education for all students and especially those with learning disabilities, Flink shares essential guidance for how to play a leading role in empowering children to succeed in school and in life. What a hopeful, optimistic book!"   —Wendy Kopp, founder of Teach for America and CEO of Teach for All

"David Flink—the most important leader of his generation in the growing movement to promote the beauty and benefits of cognitive diversity—achieves two hugely important tasks in this marvelous book. He shares the key things LD/ADHD students (and their families) need to know to meet the challenges that those who think differently most often face; and he conveys the inspiring news that these individuals should never feel alone—for they're part of a wonderfully talented and creative community, and by coming together they can grow, thrive, and love life and themselves as never before."

—Brock L. Eide, M.D., M.A., and Fernette F. Eide, M.D., authors of *The Dyslexic Advantage* and *The Mislabeled Child*

"I wish I'd read David Flink's *Thinking Differently* when my wife and I first learned our son was dyslexic; its clear and informed guidance would've spared us a lot of confusion and duress. I'm saying this not only as a parent but as a dyslexic who suffered many of the difficulties outlined in this wonderfully insightful book that strives—brilliantly at times, I should add—to shine a light on the fear and often unnecessary pain a learning disability so often results in. This book will stand out for the vigor of its insights and warm intelligence."

—Philip Schultz, author of *My Dyslexia* and winner of the Pulitzer Prize

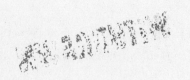

Thinking Differently

An Inspiring Guide for
Parents of Children
with Learning
Disabilities

DAVID FLINK

Fitchburg Public Library
5530 Lacy Road
Fitchburg, WI 53711

WITHDRAWN

WILLIAM MORROW
An Imprint of HarperCollins*Publishers*

To all different thinkers,
ambassadors of the possible.

To my wife, Laura,
with whom anything is possible.

THINKING DIFFERENTLY. Copyright © 2014 by David Flink. All rights reserved. Printed in the United States of America. No part of this book may be used or reproduced in any manner whatsoever without written permission except in the case of brief quotations embodied in critical articles and reviews. For information address HarperCollins Publishers, 195 Broadway, New York, NY 10007.

HarperCollins books may be purchased for educational, business, or sales promotional use. For information please e-mail the Special Markets Department at SPsales@harpercollins.com.

FIRST EDITION

Designed by Diahann Sturge

Library of Congress Cataloging-in-Publication Data has been applied for.

ISBN 978-0-06-222593-1

14 15 16 17 18   OV/RRD   10 9 8 7 6 5 4 3 2

Contents

Foreword by Harold S. Koplewicz, M.D.   ix

Introduction   xii

1. Is Something Up?   20

2. Learn the Basics   34

3. Take Action   80

4. Know How You Think   114

5. Seek Accommodations   142

6. Work Smarter   170

7. Find Your Allies   194

8. Become an Advocate   236

9. Join the Movement   254

Acknowledgments   279

Appendix   285

Further Reading   295

Index   299

Foreword

by Harold S. Koplewicz, M.D.

Writing isn't the easiest thing in the world for David Flink. He'd be the first to tell you that—he has both dyslexia and ADHD. But he has a terrific gift for storytelling. And for connecting with other people. And for doing things that look, at the outset, like they're going to be too hard. And so David wrote this book not only to tell you his own story but also to share a great deal of insight into what it feels like to have learning and attention problems.

I first met David when he was a brand-new admissions officer at Brown University, where he had been an undergraduate, and his enterprise and networking talents were already becoming apparent. That's where he started the remarkable organization he now runs, Eye to Eye, which reaches out to schoolchildren with learning and attention issues and hooks them up with college students who act as mentors.

In this book David is, in a way, offering himself as a mentor and guide to parents who are trying to understand what their kids with learning issues are going through, and how best to help them. He's frank about his own struggles and failures and successes—as well as those of many other kids he's met and mentored. He walks you through the testing-and-accommodation process in a very clear way, with lots of advice.

But what makes the book most meaningful to me (and I'd guess to many parents) is the way he uses what he's learned, often the hard way, to help the rest of us help our kids with learning issues—and, perhaps more important, to help us understand them. David doesn't like to use the words "disability" and "disorder." He thinks it's better to call dyslexia and ADHD learning "differences." And for him that's not just a euphemism: What this book is really about is how David, and the other kids he introduces us to, turned a "disability" into a "difference" by figuring out how they *could* learn effectively, instead of getting stuck on how they *couldn't*.

David's starting point is the third grade, when he overheard his teacher telling his mom that the reason he was struggling was that he was just not trying hard enough. This idea was the bane of David's young life, and he shows you how toxic that can be for kids with learning differences. One of the worst aspects of the "just try harder" approach is that it makes kids who are struggling double down on their reading or math basics—the things they're having the most trouble with—while other kids are going off to art, drama, music, and other enriching classes. It's exactly the wrong approach, David writes, because finding strengths and successes in other areas is what kids need to develop the confidence they need to tackle big struggles.

David writes movingly of how his skill at magic tricks

saved him as a child—a passion, he notes, that must have been hard for his parents to tolerate, as they worried over his rocky progress in school. Doing magic shows for kids on weekends gave him the strength to get through the week. "Magic offered a connection to other people, something I really craved as a kid who had a hard time socially," he writes. "The confidence magic gave me was absolutely priceless and, in many ways, enabled me to get through middle school."

Instead of working harder, what David wants kids to do is work smarter, and that involves figuring out how they learn best—in his case by listening to information and talking to people instead of reading. He wants kids to feel comfortable making mistakes, because trial and error is the way you discover your learning *strengths*. And he wants them, above all, to feel comfortable asking for help. As he puts it, "Mistakes are good, but asking for help is better."

David writes movingly about the many people whose help has been essential to him, and to the kids he's worked with. One of my favorite stories in the book concerns the crisis in tenth-grade biology class that led David's father, who had been a radio announcer in college, to start reading his textbooks out loud, pacing as he read, into a cassette recorder. Before David was through school he had piles of his father's cassette tapes everywhere, and to this day he carries one in his pocket as a reminder that "no challenge is too great, especially with great allies."

One thing David is especially enthusiastic about is the

fact that kids with learning issues today are much more accustomed to being open about their needs and asking for accommodations. David's first accommodation in school was a laptop computer he was allowed to use for writing assignments and to take notes in class. Since the battery lasted all of an hour and a half, he had to sit near an electrical outlet in each class. And, this being 1994, the laptop weighed in at eight pounds and was too big to fit into his backpack along with his books. The solution: two backpacks. "Having a learning disability has been described as having a monkey on your back," he writes. "I had a laptop."

The laptop made an immediate impact on David's grades, and his confidence as a student soared. But there was another consequence that was perhaps even more important, which encapsulates everything that followed, including Eye to Eye's successful programs. The laptop meant going public about his difference. I'll let David have the last word: "Since so many learning differences are hidden, making them visible can be a positive step, despite the awkwardness. Being out in the open enables students to locate their LD peers and see that they are not alone. It also makes learning differences seem less mysterious, which in turn can boost students' self-esteem as they recognize that their differences don't mean they are weird or stupid, but part of a valuable and important minority."

It's a minority David is proud to be part of, and proud to welcome other bright and talented and underrated kids into as well. We are lucky that David is here for all of our kids.

Thinking
Differently

Introduction

I THINK DIFFERENTLY

LD/A   DHD   LD/
LD/ADHD LD/ADHD LD/ADHD LD/
LD/ADHD LD/ADHD LD/ADHD LD/ADHD LD/
LD/ADHD LD/ADHD LD/ADHD LD/ADHD LD/ADHD LD/
LD/ADHD LD/   LD/ADHD LD/   LD/ADHD LD/
LD/ADHD LD/ADHD LD/ADHD LD/ADHD LD/ADHD LD/ADHD LD/
LD/ADHD LD/ADHD LD/ADHD LD/ADHD LD/ADHD LD/ADHD LD/ADHD
LD/ADHD LD/ADHD LD/AD   LD/ADHD LD/ADHD LD/ADHD LD/ADHD
LD/ADHD LD/ADHD LD/ADHD LD/ADHD LD/ADHD LD/ADHD LD/ADHD
LD/ADHD LD/ADHD LD/ADHD LD/ADHD LD/ADHD LD/ADHD LD/ADHD LD/ADHD
LD/ADHD LD/ADHD LD/ADHD LD/ADHD LD   LD/ADHD LD/ADHD LD/ADHD LD/ADHD LD/ADHD
LD/ADHD LD/ADHD LD/ADHD LD/ADHD LD/ADHD   LD/ADHD LD/ADHD LD/ADHD
LD/ADHD LD/AD   LD/ADHD LD/ADHD LD/ADHD   LD/ADHD LD/ADHD LD/ADHD LD/ADHD
LD/ADHD LD/ADHD LD/ADHD LD/ADHD LD/ADHD   LD/ADHD LD/ADHD LD/ADHD
LD/ADHD LD/ADHD LD/ADHD LD/ADHD LD/ADHD LD/ADH   LD/ADHD LD/ADHD
LD/ADHD LD/ADHD LD/ADHD LD/ADHD   LD/ADHD LD/ADHD LD/ADHD LD/A
LD/ADHD LD/ADHD   LD/ADHD LD/ADHD LD/ADH
LD/ADHD LD/

We are all the people who most often
follow our dreams, who think differently.
—Jack Horner, paleontologist, dyslexic

He must try harder," I heard Mrs. K say.

I was eavesdropping outside my third-grade classroom, sitting there on the cold linoleum floor.

These words slithered from my teacher's mouth in a tone that sounded condescending, even to my nine-year-old self. Mrs. K was a plump woman who only looked happy because her face was caked in makeup.

My mother wasn't the type of lady who wore much makeup. She was tall and thin with jet-black hair—the opposite, I thought, of Mrs. K, whose voice seemed to echo down the hallway where the other kids were listening. I tried to imagine the expression on my mother's face as Mrs. K was telling her that her son was just unteachable, and the reason I hadn't become a reader, she said, was that I wasn't trying hard enough.

I must not have been the first kid to sit in this spot because I looked over at a small patch of dust on the floor. Someone else who'd been sitting outside Mrs. K's class had drawn a frowning face there, and I traced the frown with my finger, wishing I could be friends with that someone. If he'd drawn a frown, that meant we probably had something in common: we were both failing at the one job we had—to do well in school.

When my mother finally emerged from Mrs. K's classroom, she strained to say good-bye. Something told me she was trying to stop herself from crying. She clutched her coat and purse, and as she motioned to me that it was time to go, Mrs. K repeated, "Just encourage David to try."

We drove home in silence.

After the meeting with Mrs. K, my mother and father talked to me about what she had said, and I did whatever I could to "try harder," even though I didn't really know what that meant. At this point my parents did their best to support me at home, though they always had. The school also took some simple steps to try to address my learning issues, such as placing me in the front of the classroom to help me focus.

When I reached fifth grade, they also modified my curriculum. Because I was at a Jewish day school, half the day was spent in English and half was spent in Hebrew. The Hebrew portion of the day was often a relief to me; since many of my peers wrestled with the ancient language as well, for once I didn't feel so alone.

But the school decided I would spend half the day in English, then, when my friends went to Hebrew, I would attend the exact same English class all over again. Somehow, they thought *more* was the answer. "Try harder," I was told yet again. My motivation, however, was not the problem. The wisdom in the decision to double my class time still escapes me.

The primary problem was that I couldn't read at anywhere near grade-level standards by the end of third grade and I was impulsive, by the school's measure, to a fault. By the middle of fifth grade, after numerous visits to the principal's office because of minor disciplinary infractions involving the magic tricks I adored performing in the middle of class, more failed spelling tests and lost homework assignments than we could count, and a modified curriculum, it was clear nothing was working. When my parents met with the head of the school, she recommended I leave at the end of the year. They had not done any evaluations or testing; they simply didn't know what to do with me.

Neither did my parents. They accepted that we needed to find a new school, but beyond that, they really had no idea how to deal with my struggles. Of course, very few parents *expect* their child to have a learning issue, but once it becomes clear that one may be at play, there is usually a sense of loss for what could have been. To their credit, I never got the sense that I had let my parents down, even though I knew this latest bump in the road must have been frustrating for them and even a bit daunting.

After their initial shock and disappointment, however, my parents went into high gear, and our journey began. Though they had some significant financial concerns, they chose to consider any school that was within reasonable driving distance of our home.

I had briefly attended public school as a child, mainly for the special education services that helped address my lisp. My mother knew and respected many of the teachers in the local public school, but she was reluctant to send me back to what she believed was an overtaxed and troubled system. She was also still determined that nothing was wrong with me, and that we just needed to find the right school.

One day we decided to visit the nearby Schenck School— which we didn't know specialized in learning disabilities. The head of admissions told us I'd need to be tested, and when the results told us that I was in fact dyslexic and had ADHD, I was accepted for sixth grade. When I arrived, I was overwhelmed by the camaraderie and support I felt from my teachers as well as the other kids. Not only were the teaching methods appropriate for my way of thinking (I no longer felt broken), but there were other kids just like me.

It was the most at home I had ever felt.

Dyslexia is a learning disability (LD) characterized by problems getting from the words on the page to the sounds of spoken language. Children with dyslexia struggle to learn letters and their sounds, spelling, and number facts. And when they finally start reading, they have trouble reading quickly enough to comprehend content.

They're left feeling inadequate because they can't seem

to master a fundamental life skill—reading—that their class-mates master with considerably less effort. To avoid looking "dumb" or "careless" in school, they often develop all kinds of behaviors meant to hide their difficulties with reading and language.

I also struggled in school as a result of my attention-deficit/hyperactivity disorder (ADHD), which made it tough for me to focus for extended periods. Kids with ADHD are almost always impulsive and distractible. The irony was that it wasn't hard for me to give my attention; I just gave it to *everything* and was unable to focus on any one thing.

Defining Moments

Many of you may be picking up this book at exactly the same moment in your child's life. A teacher, a principal, or a guidance counselor has told you they suspect your child has a learning disability—or perhaps you have detected this on your own. This seems to follow with being told that your child's current school just can't address his or her learning needs.

This is naturally unsettling for parents who believed they had already found the right place for their child's education. What do you do next? How do you know where to go? Many schools will provide you with direction, but many others will not.

Take heart! I'm here to let you know you have options. Though they may not be immediately apparent, today's kids with LD/ADHD enjoy a much wider array of resources than I did back in 1992. In addition to alternative/LD schools, our public school systems have also evolved, creating the space and developing the accommodations that enable different thinkers to thrive alongside their non-LD peers.

At the Schenck School, because I was finally provided with the tools that specifically addressed my learning issues, I excelled. First, the school recommended I try the ADHD medication Ritalin to sharpen my focus in class. To help me connect symbols to sounds, I was taught the Orton-Gillingham method, a phonics-based system that combines visual, auditory, and sensory approaches to language. I was also encouraged to use technology such as the Franklin Speller, a handheld electronic spell-check device. Today's kids benefit from the ubiquity of tablets and laptop computers, technology that is an essential part of any LD/ADHD toolbox.

Schenck encourages its students to move on to "mainstream" schools once they have mastered the use of accommodations and internalized the methods that help them learn best. After two years at Schenck, my academic confidence was at an all-time high, and I wanted to go where the smart kids went: one of Atlanta's most prestigious college preparatory schools. My parents let me make this important decision about my education because of my high performance at Schenck. I also believe that like many parents from immigrant communities, this was all new to them—in fact, I often was more in touch with and aware of my educational options than they were, even though I was only thirteen.

With a national reputation for excellence that appealed to me, the school I was now setting my sights on was also incredibly structured, which I thought would be good for me since things often went off the tracks when my life lacked order. Though this school did not specialize in learning differences, it did classify its students in three distinct groups: Honors, College Prep, and Transition. Because of my learning issues, shortly after I arrived, I was classified as a Transitioner. Ironically, my struggles with learning, once my only battle, became the most minor.

As the lowest members of a very clear class system, Transitioners were often singled out and bullied by students in Honors and College Prep. I, however, was doubly ostracized and faced hazing from all sides because I was one of the academically stronger Transitioners, who rather than support their fellow classmates, turned against anyone who excelled. As much as I craved knowledge and was excited to finally possess the skills to learn, the brutality of the bullying I faced broke me down. By the end of my first year, I had all A's on my report card but a failing self-image. I would gladly have traded those A's for F's to buy a little self-esteem.

My parents picked up on my misery. With my loosened school-uniform tie and half-buttoned shirt, I looked like a forty-year-old man stuck in a dead-end job. Even though there were no openings for the coming school year, the Galloway School found a spot for me. Rumor had it that the school had been built by inmates serving life sentences in a prison once located across the street.

I'd been told many times I would likely end up in jail; I wondered if my dyslexic and ADHD brothers in prison had designed the school with kids like me in mind. It seemed appropriate that I would finish my education in a school built by people the education system had failed.

The following fall, I began ninth grade at Galloway, and when I threw down my pencil, shook my head, and out of frustration said "I can't do this," my teachers didn't look annoyed with me, or turn away, or threaten me with a failing grade (failing grades, in fact, did not exist at Galloway). Instead, they replied, "Well, David, how *can* you do it?" They also helped me find new and exciting ways to help my brain learn, such as providing me with extra time on exams, squish balls to keep my hands busy during class, and a laptop to take notes with and help me stay organized. While Schenck's approach was more remedial, focusing on essential skills I had yet to learn such as reading, Galloway located the problem in the environment rather than within the student. This approach was essential to my understanding of my LD/ADHD: for the first time, I was able to really own it, and thus able to make much smarter decisions when it came to choosing colleges that were appropriate for my learning style.

Ivy Bound

I found my educational freedom at Galloway, graduating at the top of my class, and the course of my life was changed. For one thing, as I began to think about college, I was much more careful. Though Georgia Tech was a family favorite, I knew it wouldn't be a good fit for me, with its very traditional focus on math and the sciences. The overconfidence that had led me to the college prep school had also been tempered; after a quick tour of the Harvard campus, I walked away, despite the allure of its prestige. Instead, I chose Brown, where flexibility and self-direction were paramount, and I knew my learning differences would be not only accepted, but embraced.

A few days after classes started at Brown, I went to a meeting, attended by twenty-five of Brown's new students with LD/ADHD. The meeting was meant to provide us with information about accommodations and services on campus. All I could think about, though, was how few of us there were in a school of fifty-five hundred students, and how unlikely it was that we would run into one another again. I'd spent so many years feeling alone and ashamed of my dyslexia and ADHD, I now longed for a community of people who'd had similar experiences with learning but who now saw themselves through the lens of success. So at the end of the meeting, I asked everyone for their names and e-mail addresses.

"We should hang out," I told them. I received a few blank stares, a few more cautious smiles, and several phone numbers from my fellow LD/ADHDers, whose desire for community quickly morphed into a decision to help others with LD/ADHD. I became one of the founding members—and eventually the CEO—of Eye to Eye (ETE), a mentoring program for students labeled dyslexic, LD, or ADHD. Our mission was simple: to create a community of self-identified college students with learning disabilities who would mentor elementary school children with similar LDs and attention issues. We wanted the next generation of students to be empowered and know how to make their learning environments work for them while simultaneously fighting against the careless and discriminatory language of learning deficits that perpetuate stigma and low expectations for students with LD/ADHD.

As we taught our students they were not broken, we learned we weren't broken either. We gave them the same strategies to succeed we had learned on our own journeys, and we emphasized altering learning environments. Mostly, though, we just enabled them to believe in themselves and their gifts, whether it was a culinary talent, a love of math or writing, or an eye for the perfect snapshot.

The Vision of Eye to Eye

I graduated from Brown feeling as if I'd recast my fate. Everything seemed possible, not only for me, but also for the millions of kids with LD/ADHD, who, if they were anything like me, had grown up feeling lonely, stupid, and displaced in their classrooms. Two short years after graduation, I decided to expand ETE nationally—from the closet of my Brooklyn apartment.

Eye to Eye started to spread organically, as our student/mentors talked about their work in ETE's arts-based program with their peers back on their college campuses and new chapters opened every month. We now number nearly sixty chapters in twenty states and have evolved into a national movement for people with learning disabilities.

What do we do at ETE? We pair LD/ADHD college students with LD/ADHD middle schoolers in an arts-based after-school program to help them develop the social-emotional skills students need to positively change their learning environments and succeed in school and in life: self-esteem, self-awareness, and self-advocacy. Often, this is achieved simply by modeling successful and confident behavior and sharing personal experinces. In addition, we try to help kids understand how they learn best as well as how to ask for the help they need, two of the most important attributes anyone with LD/ADHD can have. Both the middle schoolers and the college students benefit from these relationships, not only academically but, even more important, emotionally.

Since founding ETE I have organized countless events for educators, parents, and students and lectured in hundreds of schools and universities nationally and internationally. I established the Young Leaders Organizing Institute to train young people to lead grassroots campaigns and advocate for their rights as learners. At every step of this journey, I have been openly proud of my mind, with all its gifts and flaws, and transparent about the steps I took to make it through school and reach my potential.

Help Is on the Way

Those insights are just some of what you'll find in *Thinking Differently,* which is part of my never-ending effort to reach as many kids with LD/ADHD as I can and help them find the same kind of success that our community members have achieved in their own lives. I know you're reading this book because you want to do the best for your child. The moment you hear your child has been diagnosed with LD/ADHD is life-altering, but it's not the end of the road. In fact, it's just a different path, and I want to eliminate or minimize some of the bumps along the way. I have seen what works, both in my own life and in the lives of everyone involved with ETE, and there's nothing I want more than to share our secrets.

What you're about to read is the result of thirty-three years in my own dyslexic/ADHD head, along with fifteen years in the trenches with my LD/ADHD brothers and sisters. In addition to outlining the steps you can take to ensure your children have full access to an education that works for how *their* brains learn, not how they're *supposed* to learn, this book is an owner's manual for deciphering LDs and ADHD. It's a manual that doesn't just tell you how to operate your brain, but how to make it fly.

Step by Step

We'll start by looking at some signs your child might have learning issues. Does your once-perky eight-year-old now cry every day before she gets on the school bus? Does your son, who excels in math, struggle to complete his reading assignments? Do the comments on your child's report cards constantly remark on his inability to sit still and remain quiet during class?

None of these scenarios confirms that LD/ADHD is present; only a valid series of well-administered tests can do that. As I'll explain in chapter 1, however, if you're seeing these kinds of behaviors, it may mean something is up, whether it's a learning issue or an emotional one. You owe it to your child to address whatever is causing the trouble.

By reading this book, you're taking an important step in understanding your child's learning differences. To help with that, in chapter 2, we'll *Learn the Basics* of LD/ADHD as well as some of the harmful myths that can hinder your child both in and out of the classroom.

My parents say they had no idea I was LD/ADHD—and my mother was a *teacher*! Yet they did know something was up and that I was not a happy student. They realized they had to *Take Action* and do everything they could to help me. That began with testing, which I'll cover in chapter 3. I believe testing is invaluable because it pinpoints where children struggle and lets parents and teachers build a comprehensive profile of children as learners to ensure they get what they need. This is essential whether you are dealing with a public or private school. In that chapter, I'll lead you through the basics of educational assessments—how to choose an evaluator, prepare your child, and discuss the results with her so that she can begin to understand how her brain learns best.

My dyslexia meant that printed text would always be a challenge for me; whenever I could (even now) I tried to access the audio version of my books. We also decided to treat my ADHD with a very small dose of Ritalin, which enabled me to make it through the school day without losing focus constantly. Without testing, not only would we have been guessing how to help me learn, but we'd also have missed my attention issues, an important part of my learning profile.

Maybe you've picked up this book in preparation for your first IEP (Individualized Education Program) meeting. You've come to the right place! In my time as chief empowerment officer of ETE, I've met and spoken with many parents who have successfully navigated the sometimes rough waters of IEPs and 504 plans. I'll share their insights in the coming pages and discuss some of your child's options—and rights— should he or she be identified as having a learning or attention issue.

To be successful, all students with LD/ADHD need to understand how they learn best. In chapter 4, I urge all different thinkers to *Know How You Think* and discuss how parents can help their children discover their brain's strengths and weaknesses. Once you know how your child's brain likes to learn, you'll be in a much better position to *Seek Accommodations*. Back when I was in school, I was able to use the latest technology—a laptop—to facilitate my learning. Today there are more and more of those kinds of options, from voice recognition software to "smart pens" that transcribe what you write directly to your computer. Many of ETE's mentors and mentees have uncovered some even more unique ways to accommodate their learning styles. In chapter 5, I'll tell their stories and help you decide which accommodations might work for your child.

Once children with LD/ADHD have the right accommodations in place for their learning style, then they'll be able to *Work Smarter*, an important piece of the LD/ADHD puzzle that we'll look at in chapter 6. But if kids with LD/ADHD don't have confidence and belief in themselves, school will continue to be a tough place for them. In chapter 7, I'll look at how important it is to *Find Your Allies*, a critical resource for every different thinker. We'll look at how to find the right ally at the right time. One day, it might be you; another day, it could be someone at your child's school. Much of what it takes to be a good ally is intuitive. But as any parent knows, there is a thin line between someone who helps just enough and someone who helps too much. It's also important to remember that allies come in all shapes and sizes—sometimes kids just need to be heard—or treated to a hot fudge sundae after a rough day.

Sometimes parents need to be more than just allies; they

also need to *Become an Advocate.* In chapter 8, I'll discuss the importance of advocacy, and how all students with LD/ADHD eventually need to learn how to advocate for themselves. By accepting their differences and being proud of how their brains work, kids will be empowered to go after whatever they need to thrive.

In the final chapter, I invite all of you to *Join the Movement.* The more people we have on our team, the greater the chance that one day, everyone will recognize all the different ways to learn and all children will be free to succeed.

Chapter 1

IS SOMETHING UP?

person person person person DYSLEXIC person person person
person ADHD person person person person DYSLEXIC person
person person person ADHD person person person person
DYSLEXIC person person person person ADHD person person
person person DYSLEXIC person person person person ADHD
person person person person DYSLEXIC person person person
person ADHD person person person person DYSLEXIC person
person person person ADHD person person person person
DYSLEXIC person person person person ADHD person person

Every Fifth Person You Meet is LD/ADHD

Life is full of challenges whether
you are learning disabled or not.
It's how you handle those challenges.
—Erin Brockovich, activist, dyslexic

t's safe to say that most parents hope they would receive the news that their kid has LD/ADHD with patience, understanding, optimism, and kindness. But despite best intentions, feelings and fears can get in the way. I understand why. Feelings and fears often arise when parents hear the words learning disability. Not exactly empowering words.

I don't believe anyone is so disabled he cannot learn. However, that is exactly what many people believe the words *learning disability* imply. While I certainly don't love *learning disability,* in order to connect kids with their rights and to a community of others who share that label, sometimes it may be necessary to use *learning disability* to describe your child's learning issue.

Most parents get very emotional when they first find out their kid has a learning disability. For young or first-time parents, the news can be devastating. Learning how to accept that your child is "different," especially when he looks like every other kid on the playground is a tall order and may take time. You may have to reorient yourself and even work through some anger as you get to a place that will enable you to become the most important advocate and ally your child will have. There is a grieving process at all levels, and you may have to let go of many of the aspirations you had for your child.

Some studies have suggested that parents often have a harder time accepting LD/ADHD than other, more visible disabilities. But just because you can't see something doesn't mean it's not equally valid and difficult to manage without some help—and it certainly shouldn't stop you from seeking early and effective intervention for your child.

At Eye to Eye, we help kids learn how to talk about their LD/ADHD, so it's not a source of shame or insecurity. As parents, you have to try your best to do the same. Remember, discovering that your child is in the company of people like Steven Spielberg certainly isn't the academic end of the road unless you make it one.

Learning that your child has LD/ADHD also opens the door to an entire community of support and hope, full of people who have not only succeeded, but excelled. At some point, you will probably need their help. Although schools may not always be as forthcoming with information as you'd like, parents who have been engaged with the system for years can be tremendous resources.

I've heard the network among parents of kids with LD/ADHD compared with the Underground Railroad. There's a ton of knowledge out there, but you have to find it. There's still a lot of secrecy about LD/ADHD and where to find the best information and guidance. In the coming chapters, not only will I let you know where to find help, I'll also provide you with insights from my own experience as someone with LD/ADHD.

Many parents want to know how to fix the problem right away.

"Unlike psychiatric disorders like depression, which can be cured, learning disabilities are not curable, even though people often do get better," explains Dr. Harold Koplewicz, director of the Child Mind Institute, a mental health resource center in New York City. "Smart parents recognize this is a long-term thing, and it's not always easy."

Even parents who have accepted their own LD/ADHD status may be saddened and frustrated when their children start to exhibit signs of learning issues. Vanessa Kirsch, who has dyslexia and now serves as founder and managing director of New Profit Inc., a national venture philanthropy fund and social innovation organization, reflects, "Until my daughter was born, I thought I was done with being dyslexic, that nothing could stand in my way. And for a while after Mirabelle was diagnosed in first grade, I still thought *we are going to ace this*." Kirsch and her husband did everything within their power to ensure that Mirabelle had access to all the resources she needed.

"We did a proactive parent search—picked a community and a school district we knew would work for us. We even hired a private tutor. Even with all the work and knowledge gained from my own past experience it was torture to see her light was still fading. I thought we had control over our resources, but we were mystified."

For some parents, the news that their child is LD/ADHD takes them by surprise. One parent I know described her son's diagnosis as "like a lightning bolt out of the blue."

"I knew he was having trouble with some of his assignments, but I just figured it was a rough patch and that he'd get through it. His vocabulary was better than most of his friends' and he was a really curious, interesting kid. So to find out he had a learning disability was shocking."

For this parent, her son's LD didn't make sense. Because he seemed bright and invested in learning, it didn't occur to her that he could also be learning disabled.

But let's get one thing straight right from the beginning:

Learning disabilities and ADHD have *nothing* to do with native intelligence.

The sooner you and your child acknowledge that very critical fact, the sooner she'll be able to embrace her different-thinking brain and all its unique potential. Now let's talk about some of the things you might be seeing that could indicate your child has a learning or attention issue.

Don't Miss the Signs

Although some learning differences and attention issues can be easy to miss, especially if the parent doesn't want to believe they're a possibility, if you're reading this book, you probably already have your suspicions, particularly if your child isn't developing at the same rate as other kids.

Perhaps your child is a bright, engaged kid who loves (fill in the blank) and (fill in the blank). Yet sometime around first or second grade, he lost some of his confidence. Maybe he became slightly shy, less willing to engage with others. Or he started to act out, getting upset over little things that never would have bothered him in the past. He may have even begun hiding in his bedroom closet to avoid going to school.

Maybe it's more like this: Your daughter, who was always first to raise her hand in kindergarten and whose gold-star homework assignments covered the refrigerator, now has a crying fit every night when it's homework time. Her little book bag is a chaotic mess of papers, pencils, and books that have yet to be read. And she's lost a bit of the light in her eyes.

If you recognize even a glimmer of your child in these descriptions, you already know *something is up*. Kids just don't change overnight for no reason (unless they've faced a recent trauma or serious difficulty in life). One possible explanation is that they no longer feel confident in school. You would probably know if they were having a great time because they'd bring at least some of that joy home with them.

Instead, school has become a struggle. But your child is

not saying anything, and you may even resist the idea that his or her struggle stems from a learning issue.

"My kid can't be LD/ADHD," you might say. "After all, I run my own business and okay, well, I didn't *love* school, but there's certainly nothing *wrong* with me, or my spouse, or any of my other kids. We'll just wait, it's a phase, his brain just needs to mature. He needs more practice."

You might be tempted to dismiss classic signs of learning and attention issues by saying "boys will be boys" or by blaming academic struggles on personality quirks such as shyness or impulsivity. While I may have acted out a bit in grammar school, I also tried as hard as I could, but it just didn't help me "overcome" my disability.

"One of the biggest mistakes parents can make is ignoring the signs, hoping they will go away," says Dr. Koplewicz. "This kind of thinking is terrible," he explains, "because kids start faking it. By sixteen, it will be nearly impossible to get the skills they need. There are holes in their knowledge because they didn't read and understand; they memorized."

As a young boy, I fooled a lot of people by memorizing my favorite books and *reciting* them rather than *reading* them. Sound familiar? As much as you want to believe everything is okay, you also need to listen to the voice in your head that says, *Hey—something's not right here.* If that's the case, the most important step you can take is to have your child tested. In the next chapter, I'll go into greater detail about many of the available options for testing. After you learn the facts about your child's learning and attention issues, you may be surprised how you feel.

"Once they finally get a diagnosis, most parents feel relief," says Koplewicz. "They understand that their child isn't lazy or lacking in intelligence, and the disability becomes real. You can explain the trajectory of their child's life. You know where the barriers are."

Reasons parents use to ignore the signs of LD/ADHD:

I don't want him to be labeled.
He just needs to try harder.
School just isn't his thing.
The school hasn't said anything and they're the experts.
I think he's just fine the way he is.

Truth is, *none* of these excuses is a good reason to avoid proper identification. What's more, your child may lose even more ground by not being identified as soon as possible. Research shows that early intervention can help develop "alternative pathways" in the brain. In other words, it's easier to shape cement before it dries. Wouldn't you want your child to have that chance?

Every kid will have to go through a period of trying different methods to find what works best for his or her learning style, but early testing can help lay out a blueprint that can be used to ensure that corrections can be made in the beginning stages of a child's education, rather than further down the line when some of a child's habits and processes have become hardwired and are tougher to change. When learning and attention issues are addressed early on, children can have good practices in place by the time academic work becomes more challenging and long periods of focus are more essential.

"A good diagnosis is essentially a prescription that says, 'This is what you need,'" explains Dr. Koplewicz. "When you don't get a prescription, you wonder how long your child can get through life without reading, how they're going to get through school, what kind of career they can have. Parents become hopeless."

Kids can begin to feel hopeless too. During primary and secondary school, I struggled to keep up with my peers and found myself spending much more time on assignments than they did. That often meant that while they were out having fun, I had to spend my afternoons and weekends catching up academically. If I had been identified as LD/ADHD earlier, I would have learned which tools I needed to become a smarter and more efficient student sooner. Other kids may have a different experience: because schoolwork is so difficult for them, they may avoid their work in favor of more enjoyable activities and fall even further behind academically.

Despite the many benefits that come from learning exactly where and how your child struggles, maybe you're avoiding testing because of the potential stigma you believe comes with the LD/ADHD label. Maybe you fear that kids are being over- or misdiagnosed and prefer not to open what you think might be a Pandora's box. But *you* will ultimately decide how to handle the information testing reveals. Wouldn't you rather know what's going on than risk compromising your child's education—and spirit?

If had known about my disabilities sooner, I would not have internalized all the subtle and none too subtle messages sent my way that told me I was stupid, lazy, and inadequate. Many of the experts I've spoken with tell me that the majority of kids who get an LD/ADHD diagnosis are comforted to know that they're *not* dumb; it's just that their learning issues make certain tasks—like reading, for example—tough for them. That knowledge makes a huge difference in how they relate to school, their peers, and their future.

Bad Reasons to Avoid Testing

I've met some parents who postpone testing because there just isn't a good time or enough time or the right time to meet with a specialist. Please remember how incredibly precious each day of learning is to a young mind. With every day that is missed or less than optimal, kids with LD/ADHD fall behind their peers and decrease their chances of academic success. In addition, the battles waged over homework assignments are usually more time-consuming than a series of tests, not to mention damaging to the mood and morale of your entire family. Don't be shortsighted when it comes to the legwork involved in getting your child diagnosed.

If you're worried that a diagnosis may separate your child from his peers and exclude him from mainstream academic and social opportunities, please know that in all likelihood he already feels separated from his peers because of the gaps in his understanding and abilities.

No matter how much effort you put into bolstering your child's self-esteem by telling him how smart he is, he will feel differently as he sits in class, unable to answer questions that other children answer with ease. Then, no matter what you say, he'll doubt it's true. But testing can let him know he's far from stupid, and he may even have special gifts in some areas.

Maybe you had a tough time in school yourself—perhaps in ways that resemble your child's current struggles. As a result, you might insist that your kid just "tough it out" and "overcome" her learning and attention issues, since you may have managed to finish school without a diagnosis or targeted academic help.

Alternately, you may be compelled to step in and do *too much* for your kid. Some parents complete their kid's homework assignments or insist that teachers reconsider low grades on their child's papers and tests. I shouldn't have to tell you that these kinds of strategies are very bad ideas. Not only do they send a terrible message to kids—namely, that they aren't able to complete work without their parents' help—but they also set a precedent that makes kids think it's the teacher's fault they're not doing well in school.

Finally, I know many families have financial limitations:

my own parents often struggled. The fees of private education evaluators can be quite prohibitive, but many practitioners offer either a sliding fee scale or financial assistance to those who qualify; insurance may cover some of the costs as well. Universities and research facilities may also provide lower-cost testing options. It can take some maneuvering, but with enough persistence, you can acquire the services and attention your child deserves. Remember also that if your child is in public school, the law requires that the school district provide a full evaluation if a disability is suspected. I will go into all this in greater detail in a later chapter.

Today's kids and their parents have many more avenues to explore for resources and knowledge than I did. It's wonderful that we have advanced so quickly—with an abundance of websites, books, support groups, and learning professionals. Now let's begin to assemble and develop your understanding of what it means to live—and thrive—in the land of learning and attention issues.

Chapter 2

LEARN THE BASICS

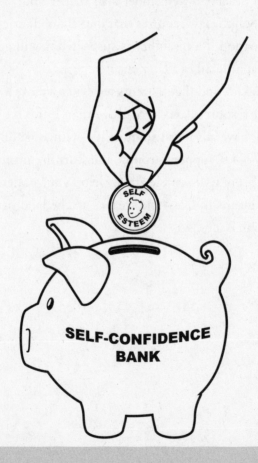

Go where you are strong.

—Paul Orfalea, entrepreneur, dyslexic/ADHD

There's a lot of misinformation out there about LD/ADHD, so it's important to dispel some of the myths and get down to the facts. First up, we need a working definition.

The phrase *learning disabilities* is generally understood to be an umbrella term for neurological difficulties in the brain's ability to receive, process, store, express, and respond to information.

This definition helps to dispel one of the biggest and most damaging myths about learning disabilities—that people with learning and attention issues are stupid. Not only is that misconception hurtful, it's also just plain wrong. In fact, people with diagnosed LD/ADHD are actually often of *above* average intelligence. According to diagnostic standards, if an individual's intellectual capacity is below normal, her difficulties are not said to stem from an LD. According to Sheldon Horowitz of the National Center for Learning Disabilities

(NCLD), "By definition, individuals with a learning disability do not struggle because of low intelligence, poor teaching, lack of motivation or other such factors. Their underachievement is unexpected and unexplained, which is why the term is often misunderstood."

It is also important to know that LD/ADHD is not caused by socioeconomic factors, age, race, gender, or parenting. That's right. You're not to blame! Letting your child eat too many jellybeans didn't cause her dyslexia or ADHD, and neither did allowing her to watch back-to-back episodes of *SpongeBob*.

What's more, the sons and daughters of doctors and lawyers are just as likely to be LD/ADHD as the kids of anyone else. As Dr. Koplewicz notes, learning and attention issues are "equal opportunity and widespread disorders." While economic advantages may enable some parents to provide their children with more targeted help *after* a diagnosis, *nothing* about parents' economic status affects whether or not their kids will be LD/ADHD.

Despite what many believe, LDs and ADHD do not occur more frequently in boys than they do in girls, even though boys may be *diagnosed* more frequently. There are a variety of reasons for this. Boys will often act out more than girls will when they are struggling in school, behavior that gets them noticed and can often start the process of identifying their learning issues sooner. Girls with LD/ADHD may also work incredibly hard to compensate for their weaknesses, which may disguise their disabilities and keep them from getting the help they need to make schoolwork more manageable.

People with LD/ADHD are not stupid, lazy, poor, mostly male, or just trying to get out of their schoolwork.

Dr. Sheldon Horowitz of the NCLD says that even now, disorders such as autism, mental illness, and visual, spatial, or hearing impairments are often confused with learning disabilities. Attention-deficit/hyperactivity disorder, or ADHD, is also not classified as an LD, though it can certainly impede learning. But though ADHD can often be treated with medication, LDs cannot.

"Many parents are disappointed there's no pill for learning disabilities," says Dr. Koplewicz, "but there's been wonderful progress with psychosocial intervention that can really help kids."

There is definitely no pill for learning disabilities, but there is also no blood test or x-ray that can predict LD/ADHD. Research is under way with brain scans and genome mapping that may produce some exciting possibilities in the future, but right now, the best way to diagnose LD/ADHD is through tests, interviews, and classroom observations.

Definitions

Learning disabilities can take many forms, and the labels have multiplied as our knowledge and understanding of learning and attention issues have increased. Terms can vary from evaluator to evaluator, from school to school, and from teacher to teacher.

I believe that all learning issues can be broken down into two main categories:

1. learning disabilities
2. attention issues

Perhaps the most familiar LD is *dyslexia,* which creates difficulty with language; poor reading, spelling, and writing skills are often symptoms. Also known as *developmental dyslexia,* it differs from *acquired dyslexia,* which is the result of a trauma or brain injury after someone has already learned to read.

Under the umbrella of developmental dyslexia, there are different varieties such as *visual, phonological, semantic* or *dysnomia,* and *mixed.*

Related LDs include *dysgraphia,* which, as the name suggests, creates trouble with written expression, while the LD *dyscalculia* makes math feel impossible to grasp. *Dyspraxia,* or *sensory processing disorder,* often creates difficulty with tasks that require motor skills, such as working with scissors or tying shoelaces. *Visual* and *auditory processing* are two other areas where children may struggle. Disabilities in these areas make it difficult to distinguish between letters or anticipate the next event in a narrative.

Dyslexia (also called developmental dyslexia)

Difficulty with language that may result in poor reading, spelling, and writing skills

TYPES

- **Visual:** Difficulty with learning words as a whole; also called dyseidetic, surface dyslexia, or dyseidesia
- **Phonological:** Inability to process sounds within words; also called dysphonetic, auditory dyslexia, or dysphonesia
- **Semantic/dysnomia:** Difficulty matching words and meanings in reading and/or speech
- **Mixed:** Combination of phonological and visual dyslexia

Acquired dyslexia

The result of a trauma or brain injury after someone has already learned to read

Dysgraphia

Difficulty with written expression

Dyscalculia

Difficulty with mathematical processes

Dyspraxia or sensory processing disorder

Difficulty with the organization, planning, and execution of physical movement

(continued)

Visual and auditory processing disorders

Difficulty in using information the senses have gathered

Attention-deficit/hyperactivity disorder (ADHD)

Difficulty with concentrating or focusing for long periods

Types

- **Inattentive:** Characterized by inability to focus, forgetfulness, disorganization
- **Impulsive:** Characterized by difficulty controlling impulses or being quiet/calm
- **Combined:** A mixture of inattentive and impulsive behaviors

Executive function disorder

Difficulty with planning and directing activities as well as controlling behavior

Confused? Fortunately, school systems and teachers often refer to dyslexia and other LDs simply as *specific learning disabilities,* or *SLDs.* Though many parents would prefer the term *dyslexia* or *learning difference,* use of such terms may limit your ability to acquire special educational services for your child. That doesn't mean you can't use *dyslexic* whenever you're not navigating the educational system; just be aware that the label SLD can be essential in certain situations to get the help your child needs.

Attention-deficit/hyperactivity disorder is an attention issue. It makes concentrating or focusing for long periods extremely challenging. It is usually divided into three types: *inattentive, impulsive,* or *combined*. Although it is not classified as a learning disability, ADHD does affect a large number of LD kids: about 60 percent of people with ADHD also have a learning disorder, while about 25 percent of those with a learning disorder also have ADHD. Many experts assert that ADHD is not actually a deficit in attention, but an inability to focus on any one thing. People who identify as ADHD will often compare their attention to the ball in a pinball machine, careening from one thought or impulse to another. It then follows that many students with LDs—and especially those with ADHD—also struggle with executive function issues. (Note: Although still used today, *ADD,* or *attention-deficit disorder,* is an older term that was used previously to describe kids who have difficulty paying attention but are not significantly impulsive or hyperactive. Today practitioners typically use the official term *ADHD,* which includes the deficits in attention identified as ADD.)

Loosely defined, *executive function* relates to impulse control, organization, switching smoothly from one task to another, and working memory, though these are just a few examples of the cognitive abilities that might be impaired.

What Causes Learning Disabilities?

The roots of LD/ADHD are very biological and are a result of an imbalance in the delicate ecosystem in the brain, which may be affected not only by genetic influences but by neurochemical disruptions as well, such as those that can occur during a difficult pregnancy or birth.

Language struggles are among the most common type of LD studied, and while researchers are not yet able to pinpoint their exact origin, they are focusing on eight different regions in the genome that might be involved in dyslexia or reading-related processes. What's more, the role of heritability in the appearance of dyslexia is as high as 74 percent.

If your child gets diagnosed with LD/ADHD, there's a very strong chance that someone else in the family has a learning or attention issue as well. My father, with his impulsive and often risk-seeking behavior, makes me think that my ADHD was shipped through his DNA to mine. Over the years, this possibility has not only helped me understand him better, but it's helped me understand myself better as well.

New technologies, such as fMRI (functional magnetic resonance imaging), have shown that the brains of those with LDs perform certain tasks differently than the brains of those without LDs do. We can see when the blood in certain regions of the brain uses more oxygen and glucose. By monitoring blood flow, we can infer which regions of the brain are active during a given task.

In non-LD readers, the area in the back of the brain becomes more active when reading; in dyslexic brains, other regions are busier. These functional variations can affect the way dyslexics process many different kinds of information, not just words and symbols.

A person whose reading portion of the brain doesn't function properly has to work harder to comprehend written material. A brain that is underactive in certain regions, can, with training, start to recruit other areas. But that doesn't mean reading will be easy for a dyslexic. Think of it like bandwidth. In dyslexic brains, reading takes up more bandwidth than it does in nondyslexic brains. As a result, comprehension slows down. For dyslexics, reading does not become an automatic activity, but rather a conscious one—and as a result is very taxing.

"The moment you introduce reading . . . the brain is moonlighting . . . it's not doing a task it was supposed to do," explains Guinevere Eden, a professor at Georgetown's Center for the Study of Learning. Unlike spoken language, reading has to be taught. Unfortunately, the ways we've chosen to teach in many of our nation's classrooms don't work for some students.

While there's a lot of great advice for parents about LD/ADHD, much of it focuses on how to "fix" children, as if they are broken or diseased. Since environments are really what predict whether students with LD/ADHD can be successful, I think we should focus on "fixing" the environment instead of "fixing" children. As soon as you adopt the "fix it" approach to LD/ADHD, you limit the opportunity kids have to develop healthy identities as learners. You also send the message that LD/ADHD can be blamed on a defective brain. This mischaracterizes the protean nature of LD/ADHD, which presents differently in different kids, for better or worse, according to environment.

Special Talents

It's becoming increasingly clear that when dyslexics and fellow LD/ADHDers engage in non-language-based skills such as graphic design or architecture, they often excel. In *The Dyslexic Advantage,* Drs. Fernette and Brock Eide argue that dyslexia is an asset in many ways, enabling dyslexics to think and reason in a broader, more holistic manner. According to the Eides, kids with dyslexia process information more in terms of the "big picture" than the details. This new and thoughtful perspective may help us begin to view all learning and atttention issues as unique and equally valuable ways to interpret the world, rather than as liabilities to be "overcome."

"Until recently, there has been little attempt to define what dyslexic brains do well," Dr. Fernette Eide explains. "When we do comprehensive testing, it's not a pattern of purely deficits; there are areas of strengths alongside areas of weakness. By only looking at what doesn't work, you're robbed of the bigger picture that will tell you the best ways of learning strategically, given the physiological challenges that exist for dyslexics."

The Eides are part of a growing number of researchers and clinicians whose goal is to reframe the way we look at dyslexia and to begin to develop better ways of teaching students who have asymmetrical processing styles.

"Until this point," says Dr. Brock Eide, "research into dyslexia has mainly focused on the way the brain handles sounds and linguistics, which was very important, especially for reading instruction. But it missed the broader picture." That "broader picture" is one that reveals a cluster of strengths and abilities in dyslexic brains that, if better understood, may vastly improve how we teach dyslexics.

Dr. Eide notes, "Some dyslexic students may actually be not just *at* grade level, but *above* grade level in terms of their ability to think about concepts, generate analogies and reason with information. It's important to know that when you've got those students in the classroom and you want to engage them and really develop their talents."

The Eides also stress that in the early years of traditional education, dyslexics can look very impaired when they are made to spend so much time on tasks that don't suit their brains, such as rote memorization of the multiplication tables. Many times, kids are removed from higher-level subjects or even subjects they enjoy so that they can spend more time in remedial classes that focus on their weak reading or math skills. The Eides believe such a narrowed curriculum is a disservice to LD/ADHD kids and can breed apathy or worse.

"Be sure not to overlook feeding the strengths for the sake of simply catching up in basic skills," says Dr. Brock Eide. "Get kids into the conceptual area sooner."

The message seems to be that if you can weather the early years of your child's education, when the focus is on learning basic academic skills such as spelling and simple arithmetic, but still take care to develop strengths and talents, kids with LD/ADHD can thrive in any arena they choose.

Attorney David Boies, who has argued some of the most important cases in U.S. history, including *Bush v. Gore* and *DOMA*, has acknowledged that he has dyslexia. Because he has trouble reading, he doesn't use scripts in the courtroom like most other lawyers do, but instead commits his points to memory. This enables him to be more flexible and make his arguments in real time, in response to what's said in the courtroom, rather than what *might* be said.

"Dyslexia is not a processing issue," Boies has said. "It's an input issue. Once you get the input in, dyslexia doesn't impair your processing, sometimes it even gives you some advantages."

Unlocking and encouraging those advantages is part of your job as a parent, so as you begin to develop your understanding of your child's learning differences, make sure you avoid seeing learning and attention issues as failures, flaws, or weaknesses and strive to view them as simply differences.

Remember: *Different* doesn't mean *less than*. It may even mean *absolutely fantastic*!

How do you unlock your child's assets? We'll talk more about that in upcoming chapters. But know that by simply paying attention to the things your kid loves to do—whether it's kicking a soccer ball, painting a moonscape, building model planes, or playing chess—you'll be on your way to helping him develop his strengths and special gifts. And since you know your child better than any teacher or expert does, you are in the best position to locate these gifts.

Many people with learning and attention issues have a tremendous amount to offer, thanks to their differently wired brains. So instead of marginalizing different thinkers, we should make knowledge more accessible to all kinds of learners. Once we remove unnecessary barriers, their brains will do their jobs as well as or even better than anyone else's brain might. They'll just do it *differently*.

Labels

Despite the label, having LD/ADHD does not mean you are unable to learn. It's just that certain ways of learning can be more difficult. If your child has a reading disability, for example, that simply means that the act of reading is difficult—but he can certainly learn in other ways, perhaps through audio-books, films, or kinesthetically.

The label *learning disability* is not empowering, nor is it even accurate. At Eye to Eye, we recognize the value the words have in the legal arena, but our focus is on building kids' self-esteem so we have started to use the term *learning difference* instead of learning disability. Although I may continue to use both terms in this book, one of my strongest goals is gaining the right to define ourselves and replace labels that hurt with those that empower.

In the end, we all can be labeled as *something* . . .

"I tell parents that the label doesn't really matter so much," says Dr. Matthew Cruger, senior director of the Learning and Development Center at the Child Mind Institute. "It's a shorthand way of describing areas of weakness and it gives prescriptions about how to address those weaknesses. But it doesn't change who the kid is to the parents."

We can all think of ways in which labels lower expectations—even *form* them at times. That is why I believe it is so important to choose our language carefully when dealing with learning differences. We should also realize that labels that get thrown at struggling students can be even more damaging than those that come with an identification.

As parents, make sure you choose labels that help, not hurt.

The Best Intentions

Sometimes even well-intentioned advocates can make choices that disempower kids rather than strengthen them. In an effort to help their students feel successful, the Hayes Street Elementary School prohibited labels they felt were demeaning. They also sought community support and mentors for their students; ETE was one of their after-school programs.

Hayes Street's school psychologist, Dr. R, was often the first to refer students to us. When eleven-year-old Phillip S sat with his mother, Kim, in Dr. R's office one afternoon, Dr. R wasted no time in getting to the purpose of the meeting.

"Ms. S, after extensive testing it appears Phillip has trouble reading." Both Kim's and Phillip's faces changed to a look the psychologist recognized. She tried to follow up her news with optimism.

"Phillip, your trouble with reading is incredibly common. Some of the brightest people the world has ever known had trouble reading—presidents, scientists, artists." Dr. R was careful to follow school policy and only use empowering language. Eventually Dr. R asked Phillip to step out in the hall. She needed to share the full scope of Phillip's diagnosis with his mother as was legally mandated.

"I am recommending that Phillip get treatment for his dyslexia. Our special education program will provide all the resources he needs to be successful. We will put him on an IEP, an Individualized Education Program, and I promise you that in no time at all Phillip will be reading just like all the other normal kids. I also recommend he join Eye to Eye, where he will get a mentor who learns just like he does, but is now a successful college student.

"One thing though," she continued. "Let's keep the dyslexic label between you and me for now. Kids don't need to carry around such weighted words as *dyslexia*."

Kim walked out and greeted Phillip with a smile, even though the words *treatment* and *normal* hung over her like a dark cloud on their walk home. Phillip had little idea what to make of the meeting, though the information they'd just received was not a shock; Phillip knew better than anyone how hard it was for him to understand his homework, especially when it involved reading and word problems. So did his mother, who spent many evenings with him at the kitchen table, trying to help him get through basic assignments.

Phillip entered the ETE art room the very next week and met his mentor, Jesse, a young college student with blue hair, a bow tie, and clothes that were black, white, and gray. Phillip, who favored sports team jerseys and baggy jeans, wondered what he might have in common with someone who dressed so strangely.

The two began an art project known as the book explosion. Instructions were simple: they could do anything they wanted to an old book to demonstrate how reading felt. Then they needed to transform the book to represent how they wished reading felt.

Jesse opened the cover of a beat-up copy of *War and Peace* and ripped out the first page. Phillip was in shock.

"Why did you do that?" the boy asked.

"You said that's how reading felt, right? The assignment is to show how it feels to read. I think we're just following instructions, no? Wanna give it a shot?"

Twenty minutes later, a third of Tolstoy's book lay in a pile.

"Well done, Phillip! I've been there—reading can be hard for me too."

Our mentors are often asked to do many things, such as help with carpool duty or support the cleaning staff (we can make a monumental mess with art projects), and we are always happy to help. However, at Hayes Street we were asked to follow the school's policy and not use any of the labels frequently associated with LD/ADHD—starting with the words *learning disability*.

If our mentors wanted to talk about a student's experience with dyslexia, they were to say they *read differently*. If they wanted to discuss ADHD, they had to use the phrase *focus differently*. When the national ETE staff sought to understand the roots of the policy, the school informed us it was part of an effort to protect children's self-esteem. While this was an unusual setup, ETE knows the importance of self-esteem, so we agreed to follow their terms.

While he worked with Phillip, Jesse chose his words carefully. "Now let's go further. How do we wish reading felt? People have told me this book is actually pretty good. How could you and I find out if that's true?"

No one had ever posed such a question to Phillip. How could he read without reading?

"If the book could just talk to me, I could listen to the words instead of reading them with my eyes, and life would be way easier."

Twenty minutes later, the spine of the book was the back of a mouth and the tips of the cover, the lips. Phillip had created a book that could talk.

As Phillip and Jesse finished turning *War and Peace* into a mouth that could read, Jesse explained that he had found books to do this for him; by listening to MP3s, he could follow along with the physical books and really understand them.

Unfortunately, over the course of the next year, students began to leave Hayes Street for safety reasons. The final straw was when a suspected gang-related murder occurred on campus. When it became clear there would not be enough students to warrant the school's operation, the remaining students were dispersed to nearby schools. Phillip would have to transfer.

Although Phillip's IEP granted the same accommodations at his new school as he had received in the past, he wasn't sure why. He knew that many students struggled with reading, but he didn't have the unifying word *dyslexia* to help him find his peers. He also lacked the word that explained that he wasn't immature or unmotivated, and that on Google would lead to the websites Bookshare or Learning Ally where he could access endless supplies of books in audio format for free.

And when many of his peers who had also struggled with reading but weren't dyslexic found their reading ability organically improve, he wouldn't know why his didn't without specialized assistance. Years later, when he joined the workforce, he'd have no idea that the ADA protected him from discrimination.

Nowhere else in ETE's work had we ever been forbidden to use the word *dyslexic*. Now we make it a policy to work only with schools that accept the words that give us many things, such as rights to accommodations and access to a community. Without the "label," Phillip was alone and wondering what was wrong with him. The choice of words is often up to adults. At ETE, we go with the word that gives kids something, even if that means they may become targets.

As parents, friends, allies, and mentors, it is our responsibility to make sure that kids with LD/ADHD feel good about something—whether it's how well they hit a baseball or how high a note they hit in choir practice. They need to be buoyed by something outside the classroom in order to survive the pitfalls of life as a student with LD/ADHD.

A Gift, Not a Liability

It may take you and your child some time to accept her new identity as someone with a learning difference, as it did for one of our ETE mentors.

"I learned how to fake it," Isaiah explained to me as we talked about his struggles in high school before he was diagnosed. "My mom would stay up with me till three in the morning to help me with homework—she even hired private tutors for me. But she did not want me to be labeled. 'You're already a black male,' she'd say. 'You don't need another label.'"

After Isaiah went off to a postgraduate year at a New England boarding school, without the support and proximity of his mother, he knew he could no longer "fake it."

"I was memorizing but not learning. Something had to change."

So he visited the disability services office and got tested. The accommodations he received helped him do well enough to gain acceptance to Middlebury College, which he enjoyed but transferred from after his freshman year. When he failed a test at his new school, Columbia University in New York, he visited its disability services office, where he learned about ETE and became one of our mentors.

"As soon as I started mentoring, my ten-year-old mentee called me out. He couldn't understand why I was so quiet about my learning issues and ADHD. And because of him— and the incredible camaraderie I felt in Eye to Eye, which became my family in college—I got through college. In the process, I learned how to own my LD/ADHD."

Isaiah's mother, too, finally accepted her son's learning differences.

"When I started giving speeches about my LD/ADHD and she saw how empowered I'd become, of course she was supportive. I told her 'This is a gift if you use it the right way, not a disability.' She realizes that now."

Today, Isaiah uses his many gifts at a charter school in Harlem, where he's had tremendous success with the students he teaches.

"Four of them are LD/ADHD. I may not be the best on content, but I am the best at showing them I care. When one of my seventh graders started with me, his highest test score was a 36. If he had to go to the bathroom, he'd sometimes just go in his pants—so he's obviously dealing with a lot more than just LD/ADHD. After some tough love from me, he now has honors in math."

Isaiah wants to work on policy and education reform, but he knows he needs to spend some time inside the school system in order to build a strong foundation and understand the challenges our schools face.

"At Eye to Eye, I learned how to talk about my disability and how to advocate for myself. Now I want to help others do that too."

As Isaiah said, learning disabilities can be gifts when you use them the right way.

Try Harder?

One mistake parents and teachers often make with children who are struggling academically is to tell them to try harder. And many do. However, that can sometimes be a bad thing. It was for me, and it turns out it is for many other kids with LD/ADHD as well, though the impact of such advice may not always be obvious.

Our ETE mentors often excel academically. Sarah did so mainly by always trying harder. As a young girl, she was called a bookworm because of the countless hours she spent in the library. But she really only spent time there because it was one of the few places she could focus. In high school, as the work became more advanced, her hours in the library grew. It wasn't until her freshman year of college, when both academic and social demands increased, that she decided to get tested and discovered she was ADHD.

Sarah's is not an unusual story, especially for girls, who are as likely as boys to have ADHD but because they are more prone to inattentive ADHD, which is less disruptive than its noisy cousin, they often go undiagnosed. Girls with ADHD also endure greater emotional distress.

Don't ignore the signs that your daughter may be struggling as a result of ADHD. Does she:

- Study harder and longer than many of her friends, often staying up late to finish assignments?

- Surround herself with dozens of books for research projects, far more than may appear necessary?

- Bounce from subject to subject during study time, never quite finishing any one assignment?

- Become visibly upset if she hits any snags in her assignments, even when they are relatively minor impediments?

Girls with ADHD may be significantly more likely to attempt suicide or injure themselves as young adults than girls who do not have ADHD, according to research published by the American Psychological Association. They also tend to develop compensatory behaviors such as perfectionism, which compels them to put in the hours to deliver strong assignments—but often at the expense of other interests and responsibilities.

"Everyone presumes that a diagnosis of ADHD is a stigma," says Dr. Patricia Quinn, author of *Understanding Girls with AD/HD* and director of the National Center for Gender Issues and ADHD in Washington, D.C. "In fact, 56 percent of the girls in [our] survey said that they felt better after finally having a name for what they felt. Only 15 percent said they felt worse. For most, it was a relief to find out they weren't lazy, crazy, or stupid."

Even without using such toxic words, well-intentioned people can still be insensitive, especially if their subtle message is *try harder.*

But as learning expert Rick Lavoie says in his F.A.T. City videos, "Learning disabilities have very little to do with motivation." It was my dyslexia, not my motivation that prevented me from being able to perform at my potential. My desire to do well meant nothing, just as the desire of someone with poor vision to see well without glasses doesn't change her visual limitation.

Yet many people with learning and attention issues keep trying to succeed without the LD/ADHD equivalent of eyeglasses. And we fail. And feel bad. And drop out of school. In fact, students with LD/ADHD drop out of high school twice as frequently as their non-LD/ADHD peers do, the highest dropout rate of any single minority group. They are also at significantly higher risk for developing the social and emotional problems that can lead to jail time or trigger suicide.

The majority of students with LD/ADHD never live to their full potential because by the time they're eighteen years old, they've received so much negative feedback on their school performance they truly believe they're "not good enough."

Self-Esteem

Most people would say that self-esteem simply means "feeling good about yourself." But that can be only for a fleeting moment, such as when you score a goal in soccer or provide the correct answer in class. The self-esteem we want to build in our children is deeper and more enduring. It has to be in order to meet the unique challenges of succeeding with LD/ADHD. Ideally, it will last a lifetime.

Rick Lavoie notes that self-esteem stems from four areas: social, competence/skill, physical, and character. Self-esteem can be derived from *innate* gifts or *created* through social capital and external input. Both pathways are essential, and both can be nurtured and developed under the thoughtful guidance of parents, teachers, and other allies.

Praise is the most important thing parents, teachers, friends, and mentors can give students who are struggling with learning. Kids need to feel good about themselves and their minds if they're going to reengage with tasks that seem impossible.

When you give kids praise, you are depositing self-esteem points or social capital that they can access when they need to. Think of it as a bank account for confidence, and if kids have enough self-esteem points, they can make withdrawals and take risks to learn new things, even if it sometimes results in disappointment. If they're bankrupt with very low self-esteem, they won't feel confident enough to ask for help and they will keep spiraling down. The goal is to keep students with LD/ADHD secure with enough social capital to fully engage with the learning process. Praise is the simplest way to keep that account growing.

No More Shame

If you are reading this, I hope you and your child are at the acceptance stage. You know LD/ADHD is real. You know it is nobody's fault that you or your kid has LD/ADHD, shy of some ancestors who have passed on genes. You also know that LD/ADHD comes with strengths and weakness depending on the learning environment.

If you are still reluctant to accept these truths, you should reconsider the facts behind the biology of LD/ADHD and the hand society has in how we view LD/ADHD. With time, you might better understand different-thinking brains and the 20 percent of folks who think outside the margins.

I have met many people with LD/ADHD who have yet to truly accept their LD—people who are often phenomenally successful. In many cases, they have learned to advocate for themselves when needed and play to their strengths and even use accommodations. But they may still live in a world of secrets and shame.

What I find most disturbing about shame is that while others inflict it, it can only persist by becoming part of a personal narrative, the story we tell ourselves about ourselves. The longer shame lives inside, the more severe the effects, like a cancer on the soul. Even the most innocuous moments can create shame, as I learned when I was a kid.

One day, my friend Kevin came over with a Superman stamp and stamp pad, which I loved immediately. I stamped

Superman on my forehead, Kevin's ankle, and every piece of paper I could get my hands on. Then, when no one was watching, my ADHD impulsivity got the better of me and I impetuously stamped Superman on the dining room wall in a polka-dot pattern while Kevin begged me to stop. But I didn't. I stamped crisscross patterns from the floor to as high as my six-year-old arm could reach. When I was done, I took a step back and looked at my masterpiece.

Then reality hit.

When Kevin left, I calculated my next step. Gathering my confidence, I brought my parents into the dining room.

"Kevin did it."

I pleaded with them not to call Kevin's parents, reminding them that he was not very popular at school. "Let's not make it worse for him," my six-year-old self reasoned.

Shockingly, my parents agreed. The shame of what I did quickly set in. Not only had I ruined our family dining room, but I had also blamed my friend, who had done nothing but share his stamp pad with me.

For the next six years, I never revealed my dark duplicitous act to my parents. Even when it kept me up at nights, I buried the urge to tell the truth. Finally, on Yom Kippur, the Jewish holiday of repenting, when I was on the cusp of becoming a teenager, I sobbed and told my parents. The wall had long since been repainted and stamp pad long since lost, but the shame had been a weight that had never left me. I learned that my parents had discerned that I had played some role in the matter, given that Kevin was a good six inches shorter than I. To this day, I am still ashamed of the stamp incident, and I learned how heavy secrets can be.

Blaming someone else for something you did *is* shameful. Learning differences are not. Ever. The shame that is incorrectly attached to them is a key reason why self-esteem is so often an issue with LD/ADHDers. But there are ways to fight back.

Self-Esteem in the Classroom

I have no doubt I never would have made it to Brown or where I am now without hard work. But I also was fortunate enough to have parents who made sure to deposit points in my self-esteem bank whenever they could. They never failed to expect greatness from me, and they never let me feel *less than*. In addition, the community at Schenck, a school that specializes in helping students with LD/ADHD, helped me develop a whole new way of thinking and learning.

When I started at Schenck, though, my old tricks were so hardwired I could not help but fall into form. On my first day, I kept getting up for tissues to avoid reading aloud, but before long, a box of Kleenex found its way to my desk, as did a squish ball to occupy my hands. At Schenck this didn't make me feel out of place at all, since the kid to the left of me was sitting on an inflated plastic ball so he could move and learn at the same time. We acknowledged each other as kindred spirits.

Schenck was built for students like me—small classes, accommodations, and differentiated instruction were the standard. At first, it was challenging to give up my old habits, but by replacing them, I gained a sense of mastery and confidence. It didn't hurt to be surrounded by other kids like me.

Reading was where I had the most to gain. As a dyslexic, I learned through phonics. Schenck tailored the teaching to my brain, which needed to explicitly understand the sound/symbol association. As we began to unlock my reading and decoding skills, I also learned how I like to learn. This metacognitive instruction has served me as well as the skill of reading itself. By trying something new, leaving old habits behind, and learning about how I learned, my self-esteem soared.

While we Schenck students loved finding out how our brains worked—that they *did* work in fact—we did not believe we were without weaknesses. I learned to read, but I remained a very slow reader. Thankfully, Schenck's teachers celebrated our use of accommodations. They didn't care how we completed a job as long as we tackled the tasks at hand.

Do your best to ensure that your child's classroom experience is helping, not hurting, her self-esteem. Since school is where most of your child's learning battles take place, it's essential that her difference is acknowledged and nourished with the proper accommodations and activities that boost her confidence.

Self-Esteem Outside the Classroom

For students with learning and attention issues, knowing how to generate a sense of worth on their own is essential to success both in and out of the classroom. Yet schools don't always provide the best opportunity to discover these inner talents; instead, the behavior that is rewarded—sitting still for hours, following directions, and so on—is counter to many LD/ADHD instincts and abilities. If schools could only recognize strengths such as kindness, curiosity, and perseverance, students with LD/ADHD would excel. Yet too frequently, the emphasis is not on those traits but on test scores and conformity.

At ETE, we are very careful not to link academic success with personal success. Instead, we provide our students with the space and support to figure out what they're good at. Then we help them create something they can be proud of—artworks and personal talismans that remind them that they are creative and unique individuals. Kids don't spend time doing things they hate; given the opportunity, they will focus on activities that make them feel good about themselves or provide some sense of mastery.

In his book *Drive*, Daniel Pink asserts that we are all

driven to achieve autonomy, mastery, and purpose in our lives. Children are no exception. Yet childhood is a time when these things can seem impossibly out of reach.

"Kids need a respite after eight hours in school, where they can't move around and carry a label all day," Dr. Koplewicz from the Child Mind Institute explained to me. "The older, successful LD/ADHD folks I speak to all talk about a family member—usually it's mom—who got them involved in something they were good at—a passion."

How does your child spend his time? What skills is he using? Which has he mastered? Even if he's playing video games or building models, be sure to praise the focus or determination such activities require. But make sure it's not empty praise, disconnected from real progress and effort. And try not to use these favored activities as carrots or sticks; let them remain safe places of comfort and competence, where life's daily challenges subside and self-confidence can flourish.

For me, magic provided that safe place. I had tried to master skateboarding, but found it lonely. It only served me, whereas magic offered a connection to other people, something I really craved as a kid who had a hard time socially. I spent hours and hours in front of the mirror doing tricks, learning perseverance and proficiency, but without the joy I saw it bring to others, I would have given up.

I got good enough that people started asking me to do shows. I'd often have three shows on Saturday and three more on Sunday, and my parents gave me enough freedom to run with my love of magic and enough support to develop it. The confidence magic gave me was absolutely priceless and, in many ways, enabled me to get through middle school.

If you let your children do what they're good at, good things will follow. Even if you don't understand their interests, as parents you have a responsibility to help your children access resources to develop and follow their passions. And if they're passionate about video games, then so be it. While we all recognize that sports and athletic pursuits are great for kids on so many levels, at the same time, what kids might learn from video games shouldn't be dismissed. Imagine if Facebook cofounder Mark Zuckerberg's parents had told him to get off the computer and play outside instead?

An ETE mother recently told me that her son with ADHD, who was obsessed with the video game Minecraft, asked her if he could start a Minecraft club at school. At first she was hesitant, but then she recognized that his impulse was really entrepreneurial—and quite typical of the ADHD mind-set. With his mother's support, Joe met with his school's principal and drew up a plan for the club, in the hopes of attracting five or six kids. Forty showed up to the first meeting—so many that they had to establish two sessions.

That success inspired Joe to work on developing a computer game of his own. A friend of his mother's who develops games for a living was impressed by Joe's plans and told the young man he'd need to come up with storyboards for all the possibilities inherent in the game. Joe has been developing those storyboards diligently for the past two years and may soon get a chance to turn his game into an app.

Support your kids' interests, even if you don't necessarily share them, and their interests will enable them to do more than you may think possible. Even if it's just pulling a few quarters out of someone's ear, the magic is in the increase in self-esteem that accompanies doing what you love.

While parents need to set up conditions in which their children can excel, it's also important to not lower the bar to ensure success. Instead, we need to provide support but be willing to let kids struggle through challenges. By stressing the effort rather than the result, we can shift the focus to process over product. On the other hand, too much praise can produce an overly competitive kid or one who is apathetic or even self-centered. You have to strike a balance.

Tough Times

Sometimes, kids with LD/ADHD can miss social cues or fail to pick up on subtle humor like sarcasm or irony. This can make relationships with their peers even more perilous than usual. Other times, self-imposed or societal pressures to excel or simply fit in can compound the anxiety that kids with LD/ADHD already battle regularly.

"Kids with learning disabilities can really feel bad about themselves, especially if they're undiagnosed," says Dr.

Koplewicz, "and that can make them anxious or demoralized and can affect their self-esteem. If they have a predisposition for anxiety or depression, it can trigger a full-blown disorder."

As I was working on this book, I received the following message through ETE's Facebook page.

> *I was first diagnosed as LD at age six. I was extremely shy and sensitive, but my teachers described me as an imaginative child with a remarkable storytelling ability. Even in kindergarten, though, I already felt different from my peers, especially when I couldn't get my letters to face the same way, hold the pencil correctly, or recall stories that were read to me.*
>
> *In elementary school I was known as the athletic kid everyone wanted on their team, which prevented some bullying. At the same time, however, I could never be the teacher when we played school because I was "too stupid" and had to deal with snickers and comments on how I went to the "stupid kid room" to meet with the learning specialist.*
>
> *In high school, I became the target of bullying after my family moved to a new area, not only because I was the new kid but also due to my learning disability. I ended up going to three different high schools because of the names I was called: stupid, special, privileged, ditzy, babied, dumb, retard,*

idiot—*to name a few. My things were stolen frequently and nasty messages via the Internet were a daily occurrence.*

One of my biggest bullies was a teacher who decided it would be fun to make the student with dyscalculia do algebra problems on the board. When I asked for help, she would reply, "Come on! This is first grade math! You should be able to do this!"

I left high school depressed and unsure of my capabilities as a student. Freshman year of college, I developed anorexia and had to take a year off to recover in a treatment center.

I am currently a senior in college with a 3.8 GPA, am well liked by my professors, volunteer in my community regularly, and look forward with confidence to graduate programs. My peers now remark, "You're so smart! How could you have an LD?," which still shows the stigma around LDs. Like most kids diagnosed LD/ADHD, I actually have a high IQ.

My road in life has not been easy, but I have met some incredible professors, tutors, and teachers who refused to give up on me. More importantly, I have a supportive family who never stopped fighting for me. I know that LD is something I have but it does not define me, nor does it set boundaries for my academic achievements. I am accomplishing things I never thought possible.

This student's story is not unique—either in its difficulty or in its triumph. There are good guys and bad guys in everyone's life. The important thing is to learn how to harness help from those who care and insulate yourself from detractors—especially if your biggest detractor is yourself.

Bullying

You don't have to have a diagnosed learning or attention issue to become the target of bullying. When kids sense any kind of difference or get even a whiff of something they can single out and mock, they will. Tall, short, fat, skinny—physical and personality traits are often just an excuse to put someone else down so you can feel superior. The problem for kids with LD/ADHD is that they often feel pretty bad about themselves already without having a teacher or group of kids throw more fuel on the fire. Their status as "different" is often amplified by their use of accommodations such as extra time or other visible learning tools.

Julie, a woman with LD I met through ETE, recently talked with me about her grammar school experience, where not only was she harassed by other kids, but by the school administration as well.

"I attended a private school with 185 students," she told me, "but I was the only one diagnosed with a learning disability. The school didn't know how to handle me so they outsourced my LD to a company that brought a mobile trailer to the parking lot of the school every day from second to sixth grade."

Julie told me that every day, the principal would get on the PA system and announce, "Julie, trailer time." She'd then be escorted to the trailer, even though she was twelve or thirteen years old. She was treated like a person who could not make her own decisions, as if she had a low IQ, when all she really needed was extra help in math. What was even worse for Julie was that the curriculum was so modified—"dumbed down," as she put it—that she ended up being behind academically her entire life.

She also became emotionally drained from the constant evaluations she had to undergo every time the school changed special ed teachers, which was frequently. She felt so stigmatized she started to fake illnesses to avoid going to school. Unfortunately, her parents didn't challenge the administration, who they thought were the specialists and knew best. Eventually Julie acted out and even became aggressive—hitting, biting, throwing chairs—in order to be heard. Then she was overmedicated until she became "a zombie," even though she didn't have ADHD.

By sixth grade, she refused to go back and demanded that her parents send her to public school. She had researched that she could spend most of her time with the general population but still get the help she needed. It wasn't until she was fifteen and finally in a class of other kids with LD/ADHD that she realized she wasn't the only person who learned differently.

Now she's a special education teacher with a master's in education, mostly because of what happened to her.

"The special needs kids I work with now are emotionally superior to us because they are so giving and only know love. When I started working with them my freshman year of high school, we had an instant connection and there was no question about what I was going to do with my future."

But it wasn't always easy; she failed her certification test seven times and had professors who told her she wasn't cut out to be a teacher.

"I knew that failing a test doesn't mean you don't know the information."

It turns out the school Julie attended has since been shut down because of how poorly it was managed. Other students I've worked with attended exclusive private schools and were also the target of bullying by students and teachers alike. Discrimination can occur anywhere: from the biggest urban public schools to the most elite and progressive academies. It can also come from where you least suspect—other LD/AD-HDers.

In the fall of 1995 when I started eighth grade at a college preparatory school in Atlanta, the social challenges I faced were intense. Schenck's classes had been held in one room, but the prep school was huge. Now I was often running a full mile to make it from one class to the next and sometimes I even got lost. More challenging than the campus were the other students. Transition students knew exactly who they were, and so did everyone else: we weren't Honors, the supersmart, and we weren't College Prep, and so we couldn't count on college. We were simply something else, the ones who didn't fit in, transitioning on a bridge to nowhere. This categorization left blood in the water, and eighth graders love the smell of blood.

It did not take long before the Honors and College Prep students discovered that I was a Transition student. No matter where I went, I was picked on both physically and verbally. Two months in and I had no one to turn to. I avoided eye contact and tried to make myself invisible.

Unfortunately, I had hit my growth spurt the summer before and I was at least six inches taller than most of my male peers. It was pretty hard to hide. The worst of the bullying occurred on the forty-five-minute bus ride back and forth to school. After a few weeks, the name calling and occasional physical abuse became more than my body and soul could withstand.

Looking for salvation, I turned to my fellow Transitioners. Many had been in the program for some time, so I hoped we could band together to create a protective shield against the abuse. Instead, the attention that had been turned on me drew the heat away from them. Not one person came to my aid.

Despite this, I was excelling in my classes—the first time I had ever received all A's. I had achieved these grades in the "stupid" class, but they were still from a very prestigious school, so I felt validated in a way I never had before. Outside the Transition program I tried to disappear, but within the program I decided to make a name for myself. I was going to be the "smart kid." I vowed that each day, my hand would be tired from raising it and my head would ache from churning out the right answers.

Bad move. As I commenced my image makeover, my Transition peers turned on me.

"Why are you trying to make us look bad?" asked Alex from math class.

"When did you become Einstein?" Rob added.

The final blow was when James, a big kid who had been held back a year, slammed his history book against my head and I dropped to the ground.

I retold my story in earnest to the principal, who assured me that folks would look out for me. But the school was huge and bullying occurred on the margins, when no one was around. I decided to suck it up, get all A's for the next five years and then bury the memories forever.

Over the summer, I reengaged with my passions—theater, dance, and magic—interests I had given up in the past year, since my peers used them to inflict further shame on me.

Fortunately, my parents recognized how miserable I had been, and that fall, we worked together and found the Galloway School, which was a much better fit for my learning style. Make sure that in addition to getting help with academics, your child has the right kind of emotional support as well. Her self-esteem is worth far more than a few A's on a report card.

Resilience Is Key

Sturdy self-esteem and resilience are key in any story of a successful person with LD/ADHD, and now we have numbers to prove it. Eye to Eye was recently selected to be a supplementary program for students with disabilities by the Wyoming Department of Education. Its goal was to improve both the dropout rate and the graduation rate for students with disabilities of all kinds through a focus on immediate academic improvement.

Because only 40 percent of all students with disabilities in Wyoming are LD/ADHD, our champion at the Wyoming DoE, Jennifer Krause, had to make a really compelling case for ETE. Fortunately, not only did we meet her expectations—we exceeded them.

Researchers measuring the impact of ETE programming on student test scores compared the test scores of three different groups: (1) typical learners without learning disabilities; (2) students with learning disabilities who attended ETE; and (3) students with learning disabilities who didn't attend ETE. The students with LD/ADHD who attended ETE scored as high or higher than the typical learners on math and verbal tests. The group that was LD/ADHD and not in ETE showed little to no improvement.

This is extraordinary because ETE did not teach a single thing that appeared on those tests. We simply gave kids the resilience and self-advocacy skills they needed to reengage with their schoolwork. But first, we helped students build self-esteem.

"When I received the test scores and learned that Eye to Eye students had made such huge academic gains," says Jen, "I was astounded. This was much more than we had hoped for. Not only was their academic improvement impressive, but they were learning how to self-advocate and celebrate that they learn differently."

Dr. Brock Eide explains one reason why programs like ETE might have such a positive impact on students' grades. Very often, he says, "we lose students by middle school . . . they become dispirited because they are no longer engaged. It's very important to keep them engaged and to look for things they do well, to feed their strengths, find areas of passion and encourage them. It makes a huge difference."

After talking to many experts on LD/ADHD for this book, from psychologists and pediatricians to teachers and learning specialists, this is the one idea they all emphasized. Help children find their passion and then support their interests. Too often, well-meaning parents and teachers will make children sacrifice their extracurricular interests or even limit time spent on academic strengths to shore up weaker subjects or skills.

Piper Otterbein, a young woman who gave an inspiring

TED talk about her LD, says that by the time she got to high school, she was done trying to overcome her dyslexia. Instead, she realized it was more important to focus on what she enjoyed, such as working in her mother's furniture store, organizing events, and volunteering. She also discovered that "my creative brain is the one that suits me best."

In college, she's finally allowed herself to drop math, foreign language, and English and instead pursue a career in design. "Work hard, eat well, and fall in love with everything," says the young woman.

For Piper, it's not so much a case of knowing her limitations as following her passions, which have enabled her self-esteem to blossom.

Chapter 3

TAKE ACTION

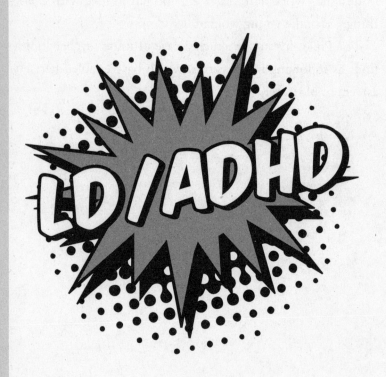

I knew I had strengths that other people didn't have. . . . My ADD brain naturally searches for better ways to doing things.

—David Neeleman, entrepreneur, ADHD

Kids with learning and attention issues don't always receive the same respect and understanding as kids with more visible challenges, so it's essential to be prepared to make a strong case when necessary. Strong cases hinge on strong evidence. Testing, and testing early, is crucial. Without a diagnosis, you may not have access to legal protections. A diagnosis also gives you leverage when you're trying to obtain everything and anything that may help your child succeed.

Let's look at how to get ready to fight the best battle you can.

Become a Learning Detective

Most parents begin tracking their child's development from birth, from snippets of baby hair to finger paintings and misshapen clay pots. As the parent of a child with LD/ADHD, you must become even more scrupulous in documenting your child's journey, especially as it relates to her education. In addition to helping you monitor progress and celebrate achievements, detailed records will be essential as you try to formulate the most effective strategy for your child's academic and personal growth.

The more you know about how your child best gathers and retains information—her learning style—the better. Is she an auditory learner, for example, learning best by listening to books rather than by reading them? Not only keep track of test results and report cards, but also take notes at teacher conferences and communicate with other parents. You want to be able to see how other factors that might be causing problems in your child's school experience, such as ineffective curricula or a distracting environment, might be playing a role as well.

If you have other children, consider the different ways they have progressed. That comparison will help you recognize the differences in development and learning style for the child in question.

The National Center for Learning Disabilities (NCLD) recommends that you collect all documents relating to your child's LD/ADHD in one place, including:

- Medical/diagnostic information

- Educational plans (Individual Education Program [IEP] or 504 accommodation plan)

- Report cards, educational assessments, and state testing results

- Communication log: copies of all e-mails and notes from meetings and teachers

- Requests for services

- Work samples

- Any other written documents pertaining to your child's education

By collecting as much information as you can on the development of your child, you'll not only get a clearer picture for yourself of her LD/ADHD, but you'll also have a dossier you can share with professionals who will be testing your child—invaluable when it comes to securing the assistance that is your right.

Know Your Rights

To receive the support provided to you by the Individuals with Disabilities Education Act (IDEA), your child must be identified as having a *specific learning disability* (SLD) that qualifies for special education services. There are fourteen categories of disability covered by the IDEA, including one called *other health impairments,* under which ADHD falls, for instance.

If your child attends a public school, you are legally entitled to a formal evaluation, also known as an *independent educational evaluation* (IEE), which consists of interviews, classroom observation, a review of your child's educational and medical history, and a series of tests. This evaluation may be initiated either by you or by the school. If your child is in a private school, the school is under no legal obligation under IDEA to provide such guidance, though some are willing to help.

In 1990, the Americans with Disabilities Act (ADA) was passed with the goal of eliminating discrimination against those with disabilities. While IDEA and another law known as Section 504 of the Rehabilitation Act protect students in grades K–12. Section 504 and the ADA protect students once they get to college, and the ADA continues to provide protection for people with disabilities on the job.

Important laws for LD/ADHDers:

- **Section 504 of the Rehabilitation Act:** A national law that protects qualified individuals from discrimination based on their disability and requires schools to make their academic programs, classes, and activities accessible to students with disabilities

- **IDEA (Individuals with Disabilities Education Act):** Governs how states and public agencies provide early intervention, special education, and related services to eligible students with disabilities

- **ADA (Americans with Disabilities Act):** Strives to ensure that no qualified person with any kind of disability is refused a job or promotion, or entry to a public-access area. ADA also applies to private and public educational institutions—ADA and 504 are the guiding regulations for ensuring equal access and opportunity for students with disabilities in postsecondary settings

- **Child Find Mandate:** Requires all school districts to identify, locate, and evaluate all children with disabilities, regardless of the severity of their disabilities

- **FAPE:** Regulation that requires "free appropriate public education" to be available to all qualified persons with a disability within the jurisdiction of a school district

Knowing your rights under these laws is essential when navigating your school system. They also represent the nexus of our understanding of LD/ADHD: on the one hand, they acknowledge that LD/ADHD is real and that those who have it should be protected by law. On the other hand, the laws also indicate an awareness that current teaching methods may not be effective and that environmental factors play a role in how—and if—our children learn.

Many of the terms used in the world of LD/ADHD are shortened to acronyms. They can be helpful to know when you are navigating the laws and guidelines for students with LD/ADHD.

Not all public schools or school districts are receptive to requests for evaluations, so you may need to make a strong case for testing. Meet with your child's teachers and school administrators as soon as you suspect LD/ADHD may be present and make use of the records and documents you've collected. These initial assessments are part of the process and will enable you, along with your child's teachers and other school staff, to begin to develop a focused plan that addresses some of the difficulties your child has displayed.

You know more about your child than anyone else does. Use that information to get the help and support you need.

"Parents are part of the team and teamwork is crucial," says Jennifer Krause of the Wyoming Department of Education. "Parents need to know that they are at the center of this team, much like a coach, and they are very much the driving force behind all decisions."

Too many parents simply defer to the educators as the experts. But you are the only real expert on your child, so trust yourself while still listening to and learning from others who can help.

Choose an Evaluator

The evaluator administers the educational assessments that will determine if your child is eligible for special services, so it's important to pick the right one. The first decision you may need to make is whether to use an evaluator recommended by the school district or to hire one independently. You might want to start with the evaluator provided by the school, implement her recommendations, and then wait to see if your child's performance improves. You can also get two evaluations and compare results or opt to avoid too much testing and just select the best evaluator you can find.

Whoever you'll be relying on most should remain accessible throughout the testing process, during intervention, and beyond to answer questions and provide guidance. Access and reliability are key. Although I once heard of an evaluator who diagnosed a child without even meeting him, not all insensitivities may be as apparent. As with your choice of any professional who assists you, do your research and follow your instincts. Here are some questions to keep in mind as you consider evaluators:

- What is her training? Does she specialize in learning and attention issues or is her practice more general?

- What kinds of tests will she be using? How will she decide which tests to use?

- Is she a good listener? Does she return your calls and is she willing to become a part of your child's "team"?

- Does she take time to learn as much about your child's home life as her school life?

- Does she have a good rapport not only with you, but with your child?

- Is she interested in communicating with your child's teachers and learning specialists?

If you have a private evaluation, you can decide whether to share the results with your child's school or not. Although private testing can cost hundreds or sometimes even thousands of dollars, your insurance company might provide coverage.

If you're working within the school system, after a series of initial assessments, you must give written consent for a formal evaluation to be conducted. *Prior written notice* (PWN) is required of all requests and before any changes to your child's learning plan can be initiated. A variety of people may be involved in this process—teachers, learning specialists, the school nurse, therapists, a psychologist or psychiatrist, and any other relevant school administrators or staff.

But the key figure in the assessment is the evaluator.

"Picking the right evaluator is more important than the measure," says Dr. Cruger of the Child Mind Institute. "Many of the evaluations used by schools are very effective, especially those for reading, language, and speech issues since the schools are already working with kids in those areas. It's the complex cases or those that don't respond to intervention that may require a deeper look."

Independent evaluators' selection of tests should be determined not only by a standardized set of protocols but also by the strengths and weaknesses your child displays both before and during the evaluation. The best assessment incorporates a combination of academic issues, information processing, attention, memory, and motor skills. The process may include questionnaires, physical tasks, and other cognitive tests that will enable the evaluator to produce a diagnosis. In fact, special services eligibility cannot be based on the results of only one procedure under IDEA.

Testing should occur over several days to offset any potential changes in mood or focus and can usually be coordinated with your child's schedule. The assessment may take place on consecutive days or over a longer period but can't take place more than once in a given time frame—usually several months—or the tests will be invalidated.

If your location limits who you are able to consult, many practitioners now offer remote services. While this option can be helpful when seeking a second opinion, it should not necessarily be your first choice for the primary evaluation because in-person meetings are usually much more productive.

Meet with the evaluator before the testing begins to make sure you are comfortable with his approach and to learn more about the testing process and how the evaluator will handle any issues that may arise, such as what he will do if your child is tired or uncommunicative. The evaluator will also ask you questions about your child and her behavior both at home and school, as well as other questions relating to her physical health and history.

You may want to consider whether or not the evaluator will be able to recommend and provide an intervention plan or if you will be referred to another practitioner. If your goal is to acquire special educational services, you'll need a diagnosis, so make sure the evaluators you are considering write diagnoses. If medication may become part of your child's intervention plan, it is important to get a sense of how the team you assemble feels about this option; those who are too quick to prescribe medications or too resistant may not offer the best care for your child.

While not everyone is willing to discuss their child's learning and attention issues, support groups and other parent forums can provide guidance. Your pediatrician is also an important resource, since he is already familiar with your child and her medical history. Pediatricians can also refer you to specialists such as psychiatrists, psychologists, neurologists, and other health-care professionals who may be able to diagnose and treat your child.

As a parent, be an active consumer. Not all evaluators or clinicians are the same. They evaluate pieces of a puzzle that must be put together to understand the whole kid—that's when the evaluation becomes more of an art than a science. In the end, though, a good evaluation should be reflective of what you already know about your child and should emphasize *both* strengths and weaknesses.

Prepare Your Child for Testing

Open, honest conversations about learning and attention issues with your child, her teachers, and other care providers are essential if you want to build a safe and productive environment in which she can thrive. Kids can be troubled by all the attention surrounding testing; to ensure a smoother path, take time to explain what's happening and demystify each step along the way.

Most kids with LD/ADHD usually know they are somehow different from their peers—it's been clear in math class when they couldn't finish a word problem as fast as other students or failed to spell their home address correctly time and time again. Acknowledge that difference, but then embrace it and let your child know that it comes with its own set of gifts, like a fantastic imagination.

A great way to position testing to your child is to tell her she's going to have the chance to explore how her brain works and how it likes to learn. Explain that everyone learns differently. Some people are visual learners, for example, while others learn best through their ears, which might also make them excellent musicians. Strengths in one area may include weaknesses in others; it's important for kids to know this is normal.

"I always tell my young patients that there are no *wrong* answers—just *their* answers, which is all I'm interested in," one evaluator told me. "These kids are so used to feeling bad around tests, it's important to let them know they can be themselves and not worry about pleasing anyone or—even worse—about results."

Here are some pretesting tips:

- Make sure your child knows the tests don't mean he's in trouble or stupid; instead, they're meant to make school and homework easier.

- Talk about how the tests aren't about getting the answers "right."

- Explain that everyone has strengths and weaknesses and the tests will show him what he's good at and also what he might need some help with.

- Promise him that the information is only for his doctors and teachers and that his privacy will be protected.

- Reinforce that the results will not change how much you love him.

Before the tests begin, you might say, "We're going to try to get to the bottom of your struggles with reading," or "We want to see if we can make it easier for you to finish your assignments without so much effort." Testing provides the opportunity to position academic struggles as part of the learning process, rather than as aberrations that are cause for shame and frustration.

Be sure to let tweens and teens know that their privacy will be respected, so they will be more likely to share their feelings. In the end, you want to send the message that together, you can tackle the tough stuff and get the help that is needed to make school—and life—better for everyone.

Try to make testing less scary by encouraging your child to think of it as a way to get to know her brain better.

The better your child becomes at understanding how her brain works and how she learns best, the better she'll be able to ask for what she needs in school, whether it's a quiet testing room or an audiobook. We know that although LD/ADHD may change somewhat over time, it doesn't disappear. Helping your child develop the skills she'll need as a young adult and beyond is yet another important way you can enable your different thinker to meet her full potential—throughout her life.

Post-test: What It All Means

Once the report has been completed, be sure to meet with the evaluator to go over the results and recommendations. If your child attends a public school and the results qualify her for special education services, the information gained during this process will guide the development of an IEP.

You'll need to understand the test results and recommendations for the IEP meeting or, if your child is in a private school, to guide the ways in which the school plans to address your child's learning issues. You may know more about accommodations than some school personnel do, so be prepared to explain why certain accommodations are needed and how to best implement them.

Schools have a legal responsibility to decide whether a child requires special education services, but they aren't necessarily all going to be adept at developing the optimal path for every student. "That's the parents' job," Dr. Cruger says.

Finally, understand that these tests, as thorough and well intentioned as they may be, are also necessarily subjective. Use the information they provide, but at the same time be cautious and circumspect. Test administration and interpretation is an art. Seek the best practitioners you can find and even then, remember that you know your child better than anyone.

If you disagree with the school district's evaluation's results, you have the right to hire an independent evaluator, though the school district may decide to hold a hearing to determine if it is responsible for paying for an additional evaluation. This may seem challenging, but remember that if you were dealing with a medical condition, you wouldn't hesitate to seek a second opinion. Don't hesitate now; you want to ensure your child gets the best help available.

Talk About the Results with Your Child

Before you tell your child the test results and what they mean, make sure you have worked through your own feelings about them. Kids need their parents to guide and potentially comfort them at this moment, not the other way around. Start with the positive. Praise the strongest elements in the evaluation and explain how those strengths can help your child tackle harder tasks.

For example, maybe it's been revealed that your son is a great auditory learner—chances are you already have an inkling of this skill, perhaps from his ability to memorize song lyrics or repeat phrases from movies. Let him know that he can use books on tape to supplement some of his school subjects and that such a talent has made him a great listener—something everyone seeks in a friend. Be creative; this is your chance to shore up your child's self-esteem before raising the more challenging aspects of his learning differences.

Most kids have heard about various kinds of learning and attention issues but don't understand how they are presented in different individuals. The language used to describe some disabilities can be dense and alienating; take time to explain each issue and how it affects school performance.

Try not to overwhelm kids with too much information, though. The most important thing is to establish an open line of communication early in the process so they know they can always come to you with questions and concerns.

Just as parents need time to accept and understand their children's diagnosis, so do children. At first, they may not know how they feel. Just as you may have longed for a "quick fix," your child may want one as well. Remain positive and encouraging about the future, but manage expectations. Most important, don't let your children think that they are somehow broken or sick. The word *disabled* is a loaded term that both parents and kids with LD/ADHD may have to work to prevent from defining them. Make sure you begin your LD/

ADHD journey in a way that acknowledges that learning and attention issues are just a part of who your child is, not the primary feature.

The label says disabled, but the reality is different—we LD/ADHDers just learn differently. So often, it's the environment that's the problem. Once kids recognize that, they are visibly relieved.

"I always tell my five-foot-five son that basketball might be a lot easier for him if he were six two," a parent shared with me. " 'But then I might not be so fast,' he quickly reminds me. 'And if you didn't have such a hard time with reading, maybe you wouldn't be such a great carpenter,' I tell him. He gets that life is full of trade-offs—and his LD/ADHD is just one of many."

What Happens Next?

If it's been determined that your child has an LD and she's in a public school, the law requires that she receive special services. Private schools aren't always bound by the same laws and make their own determinations.

In both cases, though, you'll want to familiarize yourself with the many types of accommodations and modifications that can become part of your child's education. We'll spend an entire chapter talking about specific types of accommodations. First, let's look at how to acquire them.

IEPs

Within thirty days after formal testing and a thorough review of the results and recommendations from the tester, if your child is in public school and deemed eligible for special education services, a meeting must be held with teachers, relevant school administrators, and service personnel. There, you'll discuss either an IEP or a Section 504 plan, which is slightly less rigorous in terms of its requirements and may be available to children who don't qualify for special education and related services under the IDEA.

It's essential to be well prepared for the IEP meeting. Since teachers only see your child for a portion of the day, it helps to offer information on what happens when she's *not* at school. All your research and observations will provide you with compelling reasons and evidence to make sure she receives the help she deserves. If she's going to attend the meeting as well, make sure you *both* are prepared to present your ideas and requests clearly and persuasively by discussing the testing results in advance.

Make sure you have a game plan for the IEP meeting. Take time practicing what you're going to say and make sure your child does too if she's going to participate.

"The IEP is a story about the individual child," explains Jennifer Krause of the Wyoming DoE. "It is important to include the student's strengths, weaknesses, present levels of performance, and the progress the student is making on goals. It should be extremely clear and concise for the student's next teacher, case manager, school, or whoever will be reading the IEP to know exactly how the student is progressing and what is and is not working in order to ensure progress."

Be ready to discuss your child's current educational profile, as well as reasonable goals for the school year. Then the team will consider what kinds of alterations might be made to the standard school program so that your child's needs are met.

According to the IDEA, these supplementary aids and services are intended "to enable children with disabilities to be educated with nondisabled children to the maximum extent appropriate." Aids and services may include anything from assistive technology such as a computer to specialized training for staff who work with your child to altering the way your child's progress is measured.

The IEP meeting is also the place to consider the amount of time your child will be separated from her peers for academic, nonacademic, and extracurricular activities. Under IDEA, children are entitled to learn in what is known as the least restrictive environment (LRE), which means that they must start in the general education population and if or when that doesn't suit their learning needs, only then be separated from their non-LD/ADHD peers.

As a parent, you ultimately decide whether your child should be pulled from the general population for special services. Together with the IEP team, you will also be involved in selecting state and district assessments as well as deadlines for implementation of the changes and timetables for evaluations.

You should also be aware of what the IDEA calls *special factors* for children with disabilities. They include: behavior, limited English proficiency, blindness or visual impairment, communication needs/deafness, and assistive technology.

The benefit of the accommodations offered for many of these special factors cannot be underestimated—my use of a computer in all my classes enabled me to be better organized and efficient throughout high school. Types of assistive technology continue to expand as new discoveries and uses for the most current tools increase—try to stay apprised of what's available for your child through your school's specialists as well as other parents and Internet resources. More information on special factors can be found at http://nichcy.org/schoolage/iep/meetings/special-factors.

After the meeting, by law, a copy of the IEP must be provided to parents, who must then give prior written notice before any part of the program can be implemented for the first time. Copies will also be provided to everyone involved in implementing the IEP.

Although some of the contents of the IEP may be challenging, spend the time needed to understand it so you can help implement and oversee the recommended changes to your child's educational program. Walk through the plan with your child so she knows what it means for her as well.

State guidelines can require both short- and long-term goals; an annual review of the IEP is required by law and progress can be monitored with frequent assessments and follow-up meetings with teachers and staff. Don't assume that all schools will be amenable to recommendations or even understand them; if you want your child's current school to provide the best learning environment, you may have to help them see why certain accommodations are necessary and how such accommodations enable your child to learn more easily.

Section 504 Plans

When your child does not meet the requirements of the IDEA, Section 504 of the Rehabilitation Act might enable him to receive the services he needs. Some children with ADHD may be among those who don't qualify for special services unless you show that their ADHD "substantially limits a major life activity." If you are unable to do so, a 504 plan, which is generally considered less precise and rigorous than an IEP, will still serve as a written document that outlines the details of your child's specific needs and strengths.

Much like the IEP, a 504 plan is based on collaboration between you and your child's teachers and other school professionals. Whereas the goal of IEPs is to provide corrections to challenging learning environments as well as the specialized instruction and related services certain children with diagnosed disabilities require, 504 plans assist children in seeking accommodations that will support their academic success and access to the learning environment.

If you are seeking a 504 plan, you may have to fight harder to get the right accommodations for your child in a timely and constructive manner, but you can follow the same guidelines as you would if seeking an IEP. Tracking changes and developments will help fine-tune your child's educational program and help you adjust strategies over time.

Both Section 504 and IDEA require school districts to conduct impartial hearings for parents who disagree with the school's special education team in regard to identification, evaluation, or placement of their child. Under Section 504, parents also have the opportunity to participate and obtain legal counsel.

Again, rules vary from state to state: the IDEA sets the baseline, but individual states may offer even greater protections. Contact your state's department of education for more specific guidelines.

Private School Students

Once you've pinpointed where your child's difficulties lie and learned how her current school plans to address her learning differences, you may have to make some tough decisions. Maybe you don't think the school is doing enough—or the right things—to help your child learn at her full potential.

Before you contemplate changing schools, keep in mind that all public schools receiving federal funding are required to provide free appropriate public education (FAPE) to students under the IDEA and that students have the right to receive FAPE in the school they are currently attending. So if you'd really like your child to stay at her current school, but the school district disagrees with a private evaluation or refuses to implement your requests, FAPE may enable you to seek legal recourse and get the services your child needs.

In general, most private school students do not have the same legal rights as public school students, though revisions to the IDEA in 2004 resulted in more protections. School districts are now required to consult with private schools and parents regarding every child deemed eligible through approved testing to receive special education funding and devise a "services plan," which maps out specific special education and related services.

Depending on budgets based on a spending formula outlined in the IDEA, though, the number of private school students served by the district may be limited. Under FAPE, a school may decide that it is not able to meet the needs of a student with disabilities. If for this reason the school district places a student in a private school, the student is protected by the same laws as students in public schools and the district must cover all costs.

But students enrolled in private schools *by their parents* for the purpose of receiving a more appropriate education after an evaluation *do not* have the same right to special education and related services as students enrolled in public schools. They must first acquire the school district's agreement and follow a rigid set of guidelines from the IDEA if they intend to seek reimbursement from the district. Students enrolled in private school *before* an evaluation, however, can transfer to public school to acquire an IEP as required by law.

Although the same laws may not apply to children in private schools, much of the advice is similar. Keep a complete and thorough record of your child's academic efforts, including any correspondence with teachers or other school staff. Then begin to assemble your own version of an IEP team: teachers and anyone else who has been involved with your child's welfare, such as learning specialists and psychologists, as well as your pediatrician.

Options

It's important to know the laws in your state and be prepared to request what is guaranteed by those laws. You may want to consult with a special education expert or your state's Parent Training and Information Center to learn the more subtle aspects of your state's laws and special education provisions, or perhaps even speak to an attorney familiar with education rights and procedures.

If you do find it necessary to change schools, remember

that different isn't always better. The educational requirements for teachers in private schools differ from those facing public school instructors; some private schools may have rigorous prerequisites, others may not. Make sure the schools you are considering are truly equipped to handle your child's needs. Investigate important factors such as technology and class size and realize that many private schools do not offer the flexible learning environments many students with LD/ADHD require. Others may not provide enough structure. Visit the schools and talk to instructors, students, and parents of current students for a well-rounded understanding of each school you are considering.

Charter, religious, magnet, Montessori, and Waldorf schools are some of the many options you may want to explore. Schools that address the specific learning needs of children with ADHD and/or other learning differences are also among those you may want to consider. Homeschooling is an increasingly popular option, though laws regulating it vary by state. Consult with as many people familiar with these options as you can before making a decision—and be sure to include your child during as much of this as possible.

If you decide to stay at your local public school, you can still supplement your child's education with a variety of learning interventions, clinics, and private specialists such as tutors and reading experts. In addition to looking into those paths, though, make sure you are doing everything you can both with your child's school and at home.

Get Involved with Your Child's School

The IEP meeting is one way to establish a productive work-ing relationship with the staff at your child's school. But you should also take steps to ensure that you have an open line of communication with all the most relevant professionals in your child's life, including teachers, school psychologists or nurses, guidance counselors, learning specialists, and anyone else who may be involved in your child's school experience.

Tracking your child's progress is essential and is best done with the help of her teachers and aides. Make sure you are fully aware of all homework assignments and projects and consider establishing a weekly or monthly check-in with teachers as well as between you and your child. Many schools provide online resources and homework hotlines so parents can help their children stay on top of assignments.

Occasionally, you may have to become even more involved with the details of your child's academic life. Don't hesitate to ask teachers what you can be doing at home to support your child. What may seem like too little homework to you may be part of a bigger plan by the teacher to boost your child's self-esteem or hone focus.

As mentioned earlier, one of the biggest things kids with LD/ADHD hear over and over again is that they're not trying hard enough. Making kids read *more* or *longer* is not the solution. Instead, help them figure out why they don't like reading—perhaps they just haven't found what they like to read yet. Reading can be about more than just the "great" books. It can include graphic novels, mysteries, poetry, and even song lyrics. The goal is to get kids *engaged*. This enthusiasm may then spill over into their academic studies and make a huge difference.

Some parents find the amount of homework assigned to be excessive; if you're sensing a deluge rather than a steady stream, check with your child first and her instructor next. Sometimes, assignments are missed or forgotten and pile up. Other times, teachers aren't fully aware of the volume of work students face when important projects, tests, or other life events and struggles overlap. Do your best to maintain an open and candid line of communication with teachers and aides and trust that your instincts, if not always 100 percent accurate, at least deserve to be heard.

Teachers want their students to thrive; your suggestions may even help them support *all* their students. You might want to ask if they are willing to provide models of assignments from previous years, for example, so that students can have concrete examples of what works. Many teachers are also open to breaking down large assignments into bite-sized pieces and assigning due dates along the way so students stay on track. If not, parents of children with LD/ADHD can always help them implement a similar system on their own. Students with LD/ADHD also need help prioritizing, so don't be afraid to step in and help create game plans for nightly, weekly, and monthly assignments.

Knowing how much to help your child with homework

and projects is never easy; it may take time to determine the best role to play. Different assignments also demand different kinds of assistance. You may take your child to the library or help him navigate the Internet one day, while on other days, you may have to make sure his math problems are done and history reading is under way. Formalized tools such as calendars and graphic organizers, which both you and your child review, can be the best way to monitor progress and prevent unnecessary poking and prodding.

Students with LD/ADHD often have a hard time editing their work. Reading essays and other written assignments aloud is one of the best ways to catch errors, and with current technology, it's easier than ever. Sometimes hearing a real person read an essay aloud is even better; if you have that kind of relationship with your child, you may want to help. But be careful: don't become the editor—let your child catch her errors on her own, even if she misses a few. You want to be a tool, not a crutch.

Be open about how much you work with your child with her teachers so that they're aware of your involvement. Otherwise, in-class work may bear little resemblance to homework and teachers might grow concerned about the disparity and even suspect cheating.

Not all teachers will have the experience or background that enables them to help learners with LD/ADHD thrive. If you sense that a teacher may not be providing the help your child needs, arrange a conference, and consider inviting other involved school staff such as the learning specialist or counselor.

Try to document your concerns and articulate as best you can exactly where you sense trouble; the more concrete and specific you can be, the better. Keep your emotions in check and realize that a meeting may not solve the problem. Do what you can, but then be prepared to seek alternate solutions such as changing teachers or even schools.

Other Places to Find Help

Beyond the classroom, rely on experts such as your pediatrician and other reputable professionals, as well as fellow parents of kids with LD/ADHD—and don't forget to listen to your kids themselves! I had plenty of insights on my LD/ADHD journey, and some of my greatest strides were a result of being heard by the adults around me.

The more you know about what your child thinks and feels, the better equipped you will be to help meet her needs and make sure she has the right tools to navigate the stormy seas of school and life.

Alison, an English instructor at a high school for kids with LDs, shared some thoughts with me recently as we discussed how to guide parents.

"Many times what students with LD/ADHD produce doesn't match up with their peers—or with the expectations of their parents. Learning comes from experience, from the process of *doing*. It's important to recognize that learning occurs in many places and 'dumbing down' isn't the answer. Neither is placing unreasonable demands on kids."

Alison's is a valuable insight, one that parents would be wise to heed, especially if their child with LD/ADHD has older siblings without learning issues. Learning is a process, and being too "results oriented" can be counterproductive.

The more we become aware of the prevalence of learning issues and the many ways we can help different thinkers succeed, the more solutions arise. Learning centers and reading clinics are popping up across the country to help address the gaps in our educational system. There are also some excellent private tutors out there.

In addition, a host of "alternative" interventions exist that may or may not help your child. Many of these approaches lack sound, scientific support. That doesn't mean they may not offer some relief for your child's symptoms or provide a thoughtful framework for dealing with certain aspects of LD/ADHD.

Diet and exercise, for example, are universally acknowledged to be important in the maintenance of everyone's health, not just for kids with LD/ADHD. It stands to reason that a healthy diet—one that limits sugar and caffeine intake and is based on established principles of nutrition—is a sensible tool to include in your LD/ADHD tool kit.

On the other hand, any approach that promises to "cure" LD/ADHD or calls itself a "breakthrough" or other type of quick fix isn't likely to be very effective. Learning and attention issues may shift and change somewhat over the years, but they don't go away, and effective management takes time and effort. Be a cautious consumer when it comes to your child's options. Talk to trusted professionals and even other parents before you jump into a cutting-edge study or sign up for an expensive after-school program. Your child is counting on you to be a shrewd advocate.

In the next chapter, we'll look at how to unlock one of the greatest keys to children's success: understanding how they think. The more parents know about how their children absorb new information and ideas, the more they'll be able to make sure the kids reach their potential.

Chapter 4

KNOW HOW YOU THINK

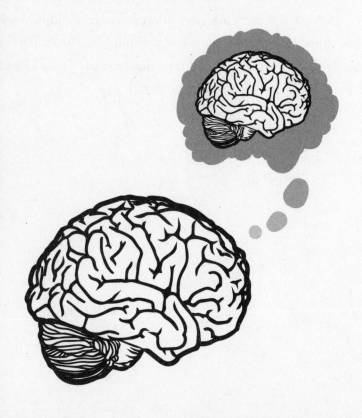

Perhaps my ability . . .
to put together different ideas
may have been affected by what
I learned to do from dyslexia.

—Dr. Carol Greider, Nobel laureate, dyslexic

Testing results provide a great deal of information to help your child get what she needs in the classroom. But just because she has a learning or attention issue doesn't mean she has a problem *thinking*. It's *learning* that presents trouble. In addition to testing, one way to help your child learn better is by understanding how she thinks—and by extension, how she learns best.

As anyone who's ever needed to get somewhere without GPS can tell you, it's essential to know north from south or at least the general direction you need to go. Knowing your brain is like having map for learning. Getting to your destination—whether it be understanding advanced calculus or finally unlocking King Lear—usually depends on how finely tuned that internal map is.

I didn't really understand Shakespeare until I watched the plays, which is fitting, since that is how the Bard intended us to experience them. Prior to college, however, I suffered through those skinny volumes just as many other students did; I might as well have been reading Greek. It was only after I *understood* and *accepted* the way my brain worked (or didn't) that I could embrace *all* the avenues (or roads, to continue our driving analogy) that could lead me to a full appreciation of the English language's greatest wordsmith.

Metacognition

Before students with LD/ADHD can take advantage of their strengths, they need to know how their minds work and how they learn best. The word we have for "knowing how your mind works" is *metacognition*. Every art project in Eye to Eye has a lesson in metacognition built into it. We ask all our students to tell us how they like to learn. If they can't answer us, we employ a variety of fun activities to uncover their preferred ways to learn. Then they're better able to seek out accommodations and create environments that are more in sync with their brains.

In our "superhero project," for example, students create their own collector's cards, featuring individual learning gifts on one side of the card and learning difficulties on the other side. For example, if you are Superman, you need to identify your kryptonite, or your weakness, whether it's interrupting people or finding the main idea in your reading homework. You also need to name the special gifts that enable you to overcome the hard stuff—your spinach, say, if you happen to be Popeye.

In the end, every student has assembled a pack of cards that includes one card from each classmate. The students then begin to see which of their classmates have strengths that could compensate for their weaknesses. Then they start forming alliances, just like the Marvel Comics Avengers, who are stronger together than they are separately. This is one of many simple strategies we have at ETE to teach kids there is more than one way to think and learn.

How can you uncover how your child's brain works? Chances are, he already has a pretty good idea, even if he's never really thought about it before. That's because we never stop using our brains, and many scientists say we have tens of thousands of individual thoughts every day! With all that activity, there is ample opportunity to observe our brains in action and look for patterns and preferences in learning styles.

You can also help your children develop greater metacognitive skills, which will enable them to be better advocates for themselves every day. Sam Chaltain, a writer and education activist, has studied what powerful learning looks like and has come up with five attributes that describe it: *challenging, engaging, relevant, supportive,* and *experiential*. None of these attributes is very surprising, but they don't always occur in traditional learning environments. The more we teach our kids how to generate these qualities in whatever they do, the closer we will be to creating learning environments in which all students can thrive.

Eye to Eye's Independent Learning Experiment is designed to uncover in a fun and nonacademic way how kids like to learn. Students choose a topic they would like to know more about—the subject can be anything and has ranged from how cows make milk to claymation videos. They can then spend time in each ETE meeting researching their topics using the school library, the Internet, or by speaking to someone—whatever works best for their brains.

Once they have finished, they are asked to present their knowledge in any format they want: PowerPoints, dioramas, sculptures, posters, models, and so on. The results are displayed for parents and friends to admire. By being able to choose their subjects, students take ownership of their education and improve their metacognitive skills by reflecting on how they actually learn. Then they take these skills into the classroom, where they can better articulate what they need as learners.

How Do You Figure Out How a Brain Works Best?

Sam Chaltain put together a great online tool called Your Learner Sketch, which can help pinpoint strengths, weaknesses, and preferred methods of learning. I hope your child already has a few metacognitive skills. If not, look back on projects in which she's excelled. What were the circumstances? Did it involve something she already had some knowledge of? What kind of knowledge? Was there hands-on learning involved or some kind of movement that grabbed her interest and held it?

If you're trying to help your child unlock her brain's best practices, look at the questions above together. You should also take note of her study habits—good and bad—to help you both recognize which ones produce the best results. Too often, parents superimpose their learning preferences on their kids—and it doesn't always work. In fact, it can backfire. So if your child actually *does* manage to get through his math homework with the radio on—and do well—then you might need to rethink your stance on silence during homework hour.

Another experiment is to set out to learn something new. Forget all the rules you've ever heard about learning: let your child do it her way. If she wants to read, let her read. If she wants to listen, let her listen. Do videos make her brain hum? Then by all means, let her watch videos to her heart's (or brain's) content, but be sure to observe the kinds of choices she makes and notice when her attention strays.

There are no accidents when it comes to learning. We don't wake up one day and suddenly understand calculus or the pluperfect tense. It takes work. But it also takes metacognition. If your child is struggling, helping her understand how she learns best is part of your job, just as it was when you helped her learn to walk.

Back then, maybe the carpet was the best place for her to test out her two feet. Perhaps you saw her take her strongest strides at the beach, where her desire to catch the seagulls outweighed her fear of falling. Her patent leather dress shoes might have been tossed aside once you saw how slippery they were compared to her sandals. Whatever worked, chances are you noticed, just as you noticed what *didn't* help her waltz across the yard with that little drunken gait that is the specialty of all two-year-olds.

What we're trying to cultivate in all our kids is the ability to monitor progress. If a student doesn't realize he's not making progress on his social studies homework, it's going to come as a shock when he fails the pop test and may result in a cycle of self-doubt and eventual disengagement. The first step in any attempt to learn something is to know whether you're learning it or not. Kids need to continually ask themselves "Do I get this?," whether it's a word problem in math or a metaphor in a novel. If they don't ask that essential question, then they won't know they need help.

The next skill children need to develop is to learn how to correct their efforts. Kids need to develop strategies to use when their standard approach isn't working. Even then, their corrections may be less than optimal. Never was this more obvious to me than during college.

Mistakes Are Good, but Asking for Help Is Better

Throughout high school, my ADHD didn't feel like as much of a liability as my dyslexia; its impact was less obvious, even absent at times. This was partly a result of the good learning environment I had at home—without siblings at home or a horde of friends to distract me, and since I came of age before cell phones, texting, and Facebook, I spent most of my days alone and relatively distraction-free.

In college, though, all that changed. Suddenly there were a million distractions and a million interesting people vying for my attention—which I gave freely and often to anyone and anything that came across my field of vision—whether that was from a desk in the library or the cluttered corner of my dorm room.

I had always struggled with deadlines, but I'd blamed my dyslexia for the sluggishness with which I completed assignments, not my distractibility. Once I faced the massive reading assignments of college-level courses, though, my ADHD procrastination techniques became a finely tuned machine.

To survive, I turned into a vampire. Every night, when my friends headed off to the bathroom to brush their teeth before bed, I'd pack up my books and march to the library, where I could finally be free of distraction. This worked for a little while, until I started sleeping through my morning classes. To correct this negative turn, by second semester of freshman year I was enrolled only in classes that began after noon, when I stood a greater chance of being awake.

At the time, both of these coping mechanisms seemed perfectly reasonable. But not only was I still not completing my assignments, I was also sleep deprived, missing out on a host of fantastic courses, and turning a shade of gray that rivaled the best Dracula impersonators.

Somehow, this is actually how I got through college. It was not pretty and I certainly wouldn't recommend it to others. I'm not sure why I didn't go back on medication, but without an invested advocate, I just used what was at my disposal. At the same time, there I was, teaching young people at ETE to think wide and far of every possible accommodation that could empower them and to have the courage to advocate for themselves. Yet I did not have that confidence myself. Because I was still doing well in my classes, I wasn't compelled to make any *real* changes.

There were a few minor metacognitive victories, however. To rely on the power of motivation and make use of my learning style, I enrolled only in compelling, small, discussion-based classes that tested through papers, projects, or presentations and I avoided large lecture courses with multiple-choice tests like a vampire avoids sunlight. By sophomore year, I made sure to include at least one independent study per semester, which allowed me to focus on subjects I cared about and learn in ways that suited my brain.

All these experiences led me to create the ETE curriculum with smart professors in the Education Department, ETE evaluations with statistics professors, and the ETE business plan with business professors. Then I really found success, as I learned on my terms by listening to books and through weekly conversations with my professors.

So it wasn't a complete fail on my part.

Part of the lesson in all this is that sometimes you don't ask for what you need until you hit rock bottom, or until there is a tremendous amount at stake. This is a shame because I bet I received some B's that could easily have been A's if only I had accessed the right accommodations. I just wasn't doing badly enough to rethink my strategy.

I think this happens to a lot of students with learning differences, especially those who manage to excel at school even without proper accommodations. Instead, their A's and B's come at the expense of a varsity team letter or a bursting photography portfolio. Or perhaps even a healthy serving of natural light.

They are usually the exception in the LD/ADHD community—the kids who when asked to jump say "how high?" Too many kids hit a concrete ceiling when they jump, and they quickly learn never to take their feet off the ground again. Instead, they give up and give in to poor grades and low self-esteem. So we must teach our kids an important but difficult thing:

Don't wait till you fail to ask for help.

For others, it's relevance that's lacking in school. Why learn algebra when you're never going to need it? Why suffer through *Moby-Dick* when all you want to do is play basketball and hang out with your friends? Dyslexic students in particular, according to Drs. Brock and Fernette Eide, need to be able to tie information into a larger framework, to know why they need to know something so that their brains can tap into their contextual processing strengths. The goals adults offer— College! A job!—are too far away and too abstract.

These promises are simply not motivational for many students. One of the reasons that ETE has been so successful is that it brings these abstractions to life—all of a sudden, kids are working side by side with a college student who's just like them—and all of a sudden, they're inspired to be more like their mentors.

Learning How to Dream

We can all inspire our kids simply by encouraging them to dream. One of our art projects encourages kids to dress up as they'd like to be seen in twenty years—a lifetime away to most eleven- and twelve-year-olds. But once we give them permission to dream, they dream big.

A young girl in Spokane, Washington, who could barely meet her mentor's eye when she began the program decided to dress up as a doctor by the third week of art room—a monumental leap of courage from a young girl who had never been encouraged to dream big. So many kids are told *they can't* so often and for so long that they start to believe it. When they're finally told *they can,* the world opens up for them in new and exciting ways.

But schools don't always show kids *how* they can. Too often, schools fail to provide strategies for learning and assume that kids will "do the work" and learn the material, but *how* to do that work is never taught. Again, metacognition is essential. To succeed academically, students need to know which methods suit the task as well as which methods work for *them.*

Expanding your French vocabulary is one thing; being able to explain the causes of the French Revolution is another. Success comes when students know how they best perform a variety of tasks: how they memorize best (written flashcards? audio flashcards?) and how they analyze best (talking through ideas? writing summaries?). In this way, the task of learning can be broken down into relevant parts that contribute to the overall goal.

Otherwise, kids often give up, thinking they've done poorly because they lack innate ability, something they don't believe they can change. It's a losing loop, a cycle of repeated underachievement. Fear of failure can result in continued failure. In fact, one study has found that kids with LD/ADHD are more likely to say that their success came from external factors and their failures were a result of poor effort or ability. This kind of thinking results in low self-esteem and the development of dysfunctional metacognitive systems, which in turn makes future failures more likely. Then kids get trapped in a negative cycle of self-doubt and even self-loathing.

To break this kind of pattern, we have to get kids to see it's not their brains that don't measure up but rather the way they're asked to use their brains that's the problem. And we have to provide them with alternatives. Accommodations provide some alternatives. But there are others as well, things that so-called natural students do instinctively, such as take effective notes, anticipate the content of exams, and learn what teachers expect in order to excel.

My Keys to Learning

Although I would hesitate to call myself a "natural" student, over the years I have learned enough about how my brain operates that I can try to control my environment for the best outcome so I can work efficiently and at my peak.

When I decided to write a book, the same LD/ADHD demons that had haunted me as a kid could easily have reappeared and told me *don't bother*. To make sure the demons stayed in their cave, I knew I needed to do everything in my power to give my brain, with all its quirks and talents, the kind of environment it needed. Because I own my LD/ADHD and am superaware of the impact it can have on anything that requires great focus and concentration (like writing my first book!), my efforts to shut off distractions and create the right environment extended beyond the garden variety walls you might erect and included all sorts of precautions.

For example, not only did I decide to take a three-month sabbatical from Eye to Eye, but I also put together David Flink.com, where I describe the book and let everyone know I'd be unavailable because I'd be writing. I also shifted all my ETE responsibilities to my staff and created an e-mail only for my "inside loop," saying good-bye to the bulk of my friends for twelve weeks.

Perhaps most important (and through the kindness of friends), I was able to line up four different places to work free of distractions: an empty office across the street from ETE, my apartment, a friend's place in the country, and most seductively, a lovely home in Colorado. Knowing that I had many options for complete solitude was a huge boon to my confidence because I realize that environment is everything.

I even purchased a very expensive (by my standards anyway) espresso machine, which I knew would get me through the dark times and address what was perhaps my biggest concern: I no longer qualified for an Adderall prescription.

Ever since college I have been able to manage my ADHD by creating environments that are conducive to the way my brain works. In my office, since I know I learn best through dialogue, we regularly hold brainstorming meetings to hash things out verbally rather than through a series of e-mails or memos. We've also established quiet rooms to work in, and all our computers come equipped with Read Please software, which can dictate anything that appears on-screen.

I try to be flexible when people want to work from home, because I know many people are more productive in their home environment. Finally, we try to practice what we preach by ensuring that our website is accessible to all learning styles and differences.

Even when I go out to dinner, I've learned to seek out the most quiet, low-key spot I can find, far from the racket at the bar and the constant stream of servers entering and exiting the kitchen, which can feel like hot needles on my brain by the end of a meal. Still, as my sabbatical approached, I grew increasingly anxious that I hadn't done enough to ensure that my ADHD wouldn't rear its busy little head.

So I made an appointment with a local psychologist to get tested. Of course, this would be the third or fourth time I'd be taking such tests and I certainly knew my ADHD hadn't gone away, so it wasn't as if I was going to learn anything new. I was just trying to get another accommodation, the same accommodation that had helped me in grammar and high school.

One night, as my nerves reached a troubling pitch, my wife, always a calming presence in my life as well as the voice of all things reasonable, said to me, "How do you find out what you need in order to think at your best?"

I stared at her with the eyes of my ten-year-old self.

"You test the environment, right?" she asked. "You haven't even started writing yet, so maybe it's a bit soon to be freaking out."

So I took her advice and just started writing. As soon as I did, I relaxed, and the words flowed out of me freely and imaginatively. This book project, after all, has been a labor of love for me, one that marries my passion for storytelling with my desire to move people and raise awareness about learning disabilities.

It makes sense that the things I'd need to write this book were not extreme or unusual. Every new environment I'm in requires some adaptation and even growth, as I stretch beyond my comfort zone. Clearly for me, the environment is one of the keys to how I think. I also thrive when I take risks, something very common for many LD/ADHDers.

Taking Risks

Parents want their kids to develop new muscles and talents. To do that, kids have to be willing to take a few risks. As someone with ADHD, I am naturally attracted to risks. So is a good portion of our population, as many studies have shown. Writing a book was a huge risk for me—I chose to leave my organization, find a writing and editing team to work with, and dig deep to uncover the stories that could really make a difference to my readers. It was a *challenge* rather than a *danger,* and as such provided a great opportunity to develop as a thinker and a person. I am lucky enough usually to know the difference between challenges and dangers, and it is my hope that all different thinkers out there see this distinction as well.

But sometimes we can't. Sometimes, what looks like a challenge is actually an insurmountable obstacle. Yes, some of us will be savvy enough to go around that obstacle, but some of us will try to scale it and fail. There is value in failure, since it can teach us many things. At some point, though, we have to be wise enough to know when a risk is worth taking and when we just need to walk away.

I'm certainly glad I didn't walk away from the many risks this book presented to me. As I describe above, I did everything in my power to line up every resource I could. In addition to making sure I had a variety of environments to work in, I also chose my allies for this project wisely. I met with several publishing houses before I chose the team that demonstrated a level of interest and passion for this project that was essential to me. Similarly, I selected other assistants to help me with the book based not only on their résumés, but on their ability to help me articulate my message and be the kind of allies I knew I would need.

I've been putting together great teams since I was in school; now in my business life, they are no less important. Everyone needs a good team behind them at some point in their lives. I've just been lucky to have access to some of the greatest players out there, whether it's my staff at ETE, my publishing team, or my friends and family who delivered late-night pizza when I was having a *Beautiful Mind* moment, scratching ideas all over the walls of my apartment.

While the story behind writing this book may contain my personal recipe for success and is a clear example of the importance of metacognition, I hope it helps you see that no matter what kind of goals your child might have, if she knows how her brain works, she'll be on her way to achieving whatever she sets her mind to.

A Happy Brain Is a Successful Brain

One of my biggest lessons in life came one summer when I set out to create a business plan for expanding ETE beyond Brown. By the end of my freshman year, I could see the tremendous opportunity ETE had to reframe learning, so I decided to stay on campus and work closely with other ETE members and professors with education, psychology, and/or business backgrounds and study how ETE could help kids and reform schools. Almost all the knowledge I uncovered was done interpersonally—through e-mails, phone calls, and interviews. I knew this was how I liked to learn and that it was crucial to honor that preference.

As a result, not only did I return that fall with a great business plan, but I also had an even better understanding of how my brain worked. Yes, Schenck and Galloway had helped me uncover many of my preferred paths to knowledge. But the business plan for ETE was unlike my other academic work; it was my passion, and represented my hopes for the future, even if I never was able to extend the program beyond Providence. That combination—intense personal investment and the ability to use my brain's assets while recognizing its weaknesses—was what enabled a kid who couldn't read until fifth grade graduate with honors and a double major from an Ivy League school.

But let me be clear: I hadn't suddenly become "smarter," nor had I "overcome" my LD/ADHD. I just recognized how I learned best, tapped into my passions, and stayed true to my values.

Perhaps the most important shift that occurred at Brown was that I finally *believed* I was smart—not because I had done well in my classes or because I was now a college graduate when I thought I'd never even get into college. Instead, I had learned I was smart from my LD/ADHD peers and from the mentees in ETE. Having a community of people who thought differently and valued one another because of those differences was priceless.

That may be what compelled me, after working briefly in an Atlanta advertising agency postgraduation, to return to Brown as an admissions officer with hopes of expanding ETE nationally. While the ETE model is very straightforward, there is complexity in the work itself. It takes training to be a good mentor; the art-based curriculum requires students to learn how to use art to add depth to the conversation. More critically, the pop-up rogue chapters that had started to appear around the country did not know how to build local community ties and were losing steam with no income to cover expenses.

So I did what I knew best, honoring how my brain worked: I went to seek the counsel of my main college adviser, who had helped launch numerous students into business success. I knew that speaking with him, rather than sitting in the library doing hours of research, was the best way for me to learn how to launch an organization I hoped would reach many, many kids.

Several meetings later, I quit my job in the admissions office. It was one of the few days in my life when I was certain I was doing what I was meant to do. (Another was the day I asked my wife to marry me.)

Although I had very little money, and knew that most small businesses fail, never mind that few nonprofits get big enough to make the change I was envisioning, I put everything aside and dove in. In July 2004, ETE's offices, which bore a shocking resemblance to my Brooklyn apartment, officially opened.

It wasn't long before the reality of my choice set in. Shortly after receiving yet another rejection from a foundation, I realized I was approaching everything too much like someone who was "normal." I had just finished listening to Teach for America founder Wendy Kopp's book when I realized that her offices were mere miles away. I was an interpersonal learner! Why was I trying to figure everything out alone in my apartment, banging my head against the wall? I googled Kopp and, with typical ADHD impulsivity, dialed the first number I saw.

"Hello?"

At six P.M. on a Friday night, my ADHD had led me to one of the most influential people in education, a woman who believed that education could change if it utilized the experiences of young people and enabled them to give back. Our meeting was the first of a dozen meetings I should not have been able to get that month, but did, such as with the head of several foundations that had previously refused to look at my applications. I traveled to Boston to meet with the CEO of the third-largest student loan company in the country, who not only made a capital investment in ETE, but subsequently joined the ETE board. I even made inroads with the heads of several of the schools helping ETE work more efficiently. I did all this because I knew I was an interpersonal learner and owned my way of functioning best in the world. Each meeting taught me more than I could ever have learned in a book or a business school class.

A decade later, I marvel at how fast it all happened. I never thought about what I *couldn't* do, but focused on what I *could* do. Instead of approaching new tasks the "traditional" way—through classes and books—I honored how my brain worked and learned how to write a business plan directly from a professor and sought advice in face-to-face meetings rather than by e-mail.

All the hardships I had experienced in my education taught me what I could handle on my own and when I would need help. I saw that asking for donations was no different from asking for extra time on a test and writing a good paper was no different from writing a good book or a good grant, as long as I was willing to get a good editor.

These kinds of skills—knowing how your brain works, when to ask for help, and making sure to get the kind of help you need—are essential for the success not just of students with LD/ADHD, but for all of us. As parents, we just need to make sure our kids develop these habits as soon as they can.

Creative Problem Solving

What I'm saying in this chapter is not a revelation for many people with learning differences. Many LD/ADHDers often figure out how they learn best as soon as they hit an obstacle, which can force them to problem-solve creatively. That may be one of the numerous reasons why so many successful entrepreneurs and business luminaries are LD/ADHD: they *had* to come up with a better way, because traditional methods of problem solving just didn't work for them.

Paul Orfalea, founder of Kinko's, is just such an example. Dyslexic and ADHD, Orfalea couldn't do things like everyone else—both reading and focusing for long periods were exceptionally difficult for him. What he could do instead was uncover alternate solutions and develop great relationships—

the building blocks for a business with revenues of over two billion dollars a year.

Orfalea calls learning and attention issues "learning opportunities." His own difficulties with reading made him a poor note taker in college, so he organized study groups with friends who could share ideas from class with him verbally, which was his preferred way to learn. He provided pizza and beer—and photocopies of everyone's notes. Not only did that experience give rise to a unique business idea, but he also learned to surround himself with people who had complementary skill sets to his own—not unlike what we try to teach our mentees at ETE.

Orfalea ended up building a company famous for how well it treats its employees. Even though he may lack many of the skill other CEOs take for granted, Orfalea has plenty of allies and relies on them to handle what he can't while he focuses on broader ideas and problem solving.

Clearly, that's been a recipe for success.

An essential ingredient in everyone's recipe for success should be self-knowledge. Most successful people—at least the ones who've had to struggle a bit, and that usually means us different thinkers—cultivate such awareness, since it can only lead to wiser decisions and better outcomes. Since the seat of a different thinker's difference lies in the brain, then it only makes sense to begin there and try to unlock what makes it different as well as what makes it happy.

High-Stakes Testing

All these strategies revolve not around results but around the learning *process*. If we can make that process more transparent and accessible for all students, then everyone will have a better chance at understanding and succeeding.

That said, the increased reliance on high-stakes testing—the kind of testing that has important consequences for a student's future—isn't good news for any of our kids. We can only hope that, with time, we will find our way past such reductive attempts to quantify what's working and what isn't. In the meantime, however, we need to make sure our kids with LD/ADHD have everything they need to enable their performance to meet—and even exceed—their potential.

What are some of the ways we can do this? As I outlined in chapter 3, get a solid diagnosis to access proper accommodations, whether it be extra time, extra breaks, or use of a computer. Next, make sure your child understands that rather than measuring innate ability, standardized tests simply reflect how well students take these tests. Just as a golf score can't predict how well you'd do on a slalom course, neither can a multiple-choice math exam predict how well you will do in life—or even on a book report.

Finally, we have to let the cat out of the bag. All the test preparation companies have already done so, even as they manage to package the same information in ten dozen different ways. What these companies realized long ago is that to help kids raise their scores, all they needed to do was map out what good test takers do intuitively—use simple, clear, and logical steps that demystify learning and test taking and open them up to anyone who wants to *try*.

This approach can extend beyond standardized tests, and it's something you can do at home without the help of expensive tutoring. It's more important to be a good thinker than a good student. Good students may get high grades, but good thinkers find success in whatever they set their minds to.

Everyone can think. Once we recognize that, the world is ours to unlock. In the next chapter, we'll look at specific ways to help children unlock their true potential in the classroom through accommodations, another key to learning.

Chapter 5

SEEK ACCOMMODATIONS

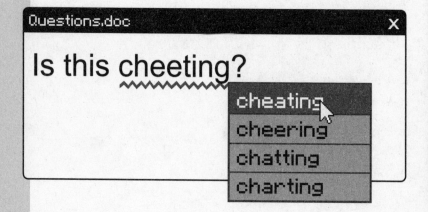

If you have kids who are struggling with dyslexia, the greatest gift you can give them is the sense that nothing is unattainable.

—Orlando Bloom, actor, dyslexic

Both testing and understanding how your child thinks will guide you toward the right accommodations, an essential piece of the learning puzzle for children with learning differences.

According to the National Center for Learning Disabilities, accommodations are "alterations in the way tasks are presented that allow children with learning disabilities to complete the same assignments as other students. Accommodations do not alter the content of assignments, give students an unfair advantage or in the case of assessments, change what a test measures. They do make it possible for students with LD/ADHD to show what they know without being impeded by their disability."

Alterations in setting, timing, scheduling, and response type may begin to address some of your child's learning differences. Any reasonable option should be considered as you brainstorm ideas to make learning more accessible for your different thinker.

A Wide Range of Possibilities

Many things that help students learn can be seen as accommodations, from the simple, such as preferential seating in the front of a classroom, to the more complex, such as a state-of-the-art computer program.

Extra time on tests is one of the most common accommodations for the 85 percent of elementary or middle school children with learning and attention issues in language arts classes. Other alterations include modified assignments or tests; more frequent feedback; access to books in audio format; use of computers, readers, or other types of assistants; and slower-paced instruction.

Not all accommodations are created equal. Beware of those that are just handed out or randomly assigned—one-size-fits-all accommodations are just as problematic as one-size-fits-all learning environments.

Let's say that one year your child is allowed extra time on tests, which provides tremendous assistance. But the following year, due to an increase in the number and length of written assignments, the use of a computer during essay tests to help with spelling and legibility may also become a necessity. Children's learning needs often change over time, and their learning plans should always be a reflection of those needs.

Again, the importance of a good evaluation is clear: with proper testing and diagnosis, effective accommodations are easier to locate. What's more, without a diagnosis, proper accommodations may be difficult to acquire.

You and your child are the best judges of the effectiveness of specific accommodations. Although teachers are required to sign their students' IEPs, that doesn't mean they've always had the chance to read and understand every element. The more communicative you can be about your child's needs, the greater the chance teachers will appreciate and implement accommodations correctly. While teachers are responsible for many kids, you are responsible only for your own.

Activities that help your child out of the classroom may be key to finding the right accommodations in the classroom. One ETE child saw great benefits from therapeutic woodworking. When his mother shared this information in his IEP meeting, everyone was able to recognize that hands-on, active learning helped her son learn better. Don't be afraid to suggest accommodations that might not be at the top of one's mind; sometimes your insights will start a conversation that leads to a better learning environment.

Altering the environment to suit learning needs is exactly what good accommodations set out to do. If your child is dyslexic, audiobooks may be the key in dealing with assignments that require reading. If she needs to focus despite her ADHD in order to perform well on a test, but she's sitting next to someone who is tapping his pencil constantly, she should take the test in a quiet, distraction-free environment.

We all make changes similar to these every day and rarely think of them as disability fixes, but rather as life enhancements or conveniences. People who have a hard time with directions no longer struggle as much because of GPS on smartphones. And folks with bad handwriting are saved from embarrassment by computers and e-mail. These are both accommodations for life's challenges. Kids with LD/ADHD just need a little extra help finding the right accommodations for their particular challenges.

Sometimes the best accommodations are also the most unique. I know a young baseball player who actually processes new information better when he's throwing a ball against his bedroom wall. Another student is less distracted when there's background music on as he studies, and a young woman who worked with me sings while she writes.

Though some parents may find these behaviors strange at first—even annoying—if students perform better because of a quirky habit or two, as long as no one's getting hurt, the wisest path may be to let different thinkers do whatever it takes for their brains to work best. You'll know if it's an effective change if their performance improves. If it doesn't—or if their quirky habit makes things worse—then you'll need to work with your child to find better solutions.

If you've ever solved a pressing dilemma on a long drive, or come up with a creative solution as you were mowing the lawn, it shouldn't be hard to imagine that critical thinking can be activated by seemingly unrelated activities. It's not a big leap to realize that unconventional behaviors might help some students learn better. Coping mechanisms that may seem odd to us may only be a response to a very restricted definition of the "right way" to learn.

Accommodations free us from preconceptions about how to learn and enable different thinkers not only to meet their potential, but to thrive.

Traditional Versus Asset-Based Accommodations

There's a distinction between *traditional* accommodations, which alter the learning environment in ways that work for many different kinds of students, and *asset-based* accommodations, which look to each student's specific strengths to make constructive changes to the learning process.

Traditional, or "straight," accommodations can be easier to acquire and more readily accepted than less common types of alterations. Extra time on tests, for example, is often essential for dyslexics and students with processing issues who need the time to read, retrieve, and comprehend and is a very common alteration.

As Dr. Sally Shaywitz of the Yale Center for Creativity and Dyslexia explains, "Dyslexia robs a person of time . . .

accommodations like extra time return part of it . . . a person who is dyslexic has as much a physiologic need for extra time as a diabetic has a need for insulin."

The way some students with LD/ADHD struggle to finish assignments at the same pace as their non-LD/ADHD peers makes their need for extra time obvious, just as it's clear why a hearing aid helps someone who can't hear. The accommodation fits the deficit. But such fixes aren't always so apparent. What's more, what works for one kind of learning difference may actually pose a problem for others.

For kids with ADHD, for example, extra time on tests might just give them more time to deliberate between two answers, get distracted by the pattern of ceiling tiles, or go off on a tangent when writing an in-class essay. Better solutions for their needs might include extra breaks or allowing them to take tests alone in a room so there are no distractions.

Asset-based accommodations, which rely on a student's strengths, can often be the optimal way to ensure peak performance. For example, if a child learns best by talking over her ideas and insights rather than by memorizing formulas for multiple-choice exams, then testing her orally would be ideal. Many kids are *kinesthetic learners,* which means they learn best by doing, so activities that engage their hands as well as their minds are often the best way to help them learn.

There will probably be a trial-and-error period as you discover which tools provide the most assistance. As soon as you suspect one may help, practice it at home with your child, since kids can feel pressured and anxious when they are in the classroom. The goal is to make an accommodation feel like a seamless part of children's education, something that enables them to compete with their peers and display all their unique talents.

My First Accommodation

Even successful accommodations can pose challenges. Kids who already stand out from the crowd can become even more visible, and this carries its own risks, something I learned as a high school student back in 1994.

Before I began my first year at Galloway, the administration asked my parents to purchase a laptop for me since they knew I had learning issues and that a laptop would help me with organization, spelling, and note taking. It was an unusual request; few people in 1994 had laptops, and if they did, kids rarely brought them to school. Money was tight at the time because my father was starting a new business, but my parents were committed. My father, a CEO and entrepreneur, didn't have a laptop, but his fourteen-year-old son would have one.

We walked out of Office Depot with what was essentially an eight-pound electronic typewriter with a built-in spell-checker. When I got home and put it on my desk, I stared at it from across the room. The cardboard IBM box housed many things: a tremendous gift and gesture of faith in my education from my parents; a debt that my parents would be paying off in twenty-four installments; and the opportunity for me never again to worry about turning in a paper with spelling errors. I would also finally be able to read my notes after class and not lose my work. That night, I stayed up late trying to learn my way around my latest accommodation. It was not until the morning when two big problems occurred to me.

First, the battery of my new IBM ThinkPad lasted a whopping hour and a half, tops. How was I supposed to use it in all my classes if it would run out of juice long before lunchtime? Second, the thing was huge. If I put it in my backpack, there was no room for books. I was already worried about standing out, and walking around with a suitcase (this was before the era of laptop bags) would not be conducive to blending in.

So instead I took two backpacks, one for my books and one for my computer. Something told me that two backpacks made for a slightly smaller bull's-eye than a big suitcase. Having a learning disability has been described as having a monkey on your back. I had a laptop.

I tossed and turned the night before my first day. How was I going to explain to my teachers and peers why I had two backpacks and that I'd have to always sit near a power outlet so my accommodation didn't run out of juice? *Accommodation*—an odd word to find in a fourteen-year-old's vocabulary and yet I knew it intimately.

My first class was English with Mr. V, a new teacher. I

mustered up my confidence and approached him to explain myself. He greeted me with a friendly "Hello, David."

"Hello, Mr. V." I paused as I tried to figure out how he knew who I was and searched for my next words.

"There are power outlets over there and over there. If I catch you playing solitaire, the computer is mine. Got it?" He smiled at me warmly. I said thanks and sat down near one of the outlets. My mind was racing.

What had just happened? The teachers had clearly been informed I would be using a laptop in their classes. Instead of singling me out as I feared it would, I suddenly had a symbol that proved I wasn't faking. After all, no family would be so insane as to purchase a laptop for their kid if dyslexia wasn't *real*.

My brain shot to Mrs. K: *If David would only try harder.* My new school and teacher already understood that I was ready to try hard. And it was clear that my family had my back to invest so much in me.

In fact, all my teachers knew that the kid with two backpacks needed a power outlet and that the laptop would make all our jobs easier. This was thanks to my mother, who had met with my instructors to go over the details of my learning plan before school began. She still let me prepare for my first attempt at an explanation with Mr. V, a watershed moment in my identity as a student, but the path had been smoothed somewhat by her efforts.

Several months later, I received some of the best grades I had ever achieved.

Having two backpacks and a computer did make me stick out a little more, but even this had its upside: it helped my teachers better understand how to teach me and what I needed to succeed. My confidence as a student soared—and the second backpack didn't turn out to be that cumbersome after all.

Out in the Open

My laptop had both pros and cons; while it visibly legitimized my learning issues, making it easier for people to help me and enabling me to organize my notes and thoughts, it also announced my difference, even when I may have wished to remain anonymous. In the end, though, I was able to more confidently interact with my LD/ADHD rather than have to think of it as some shameful personal failing.

Since so many learning differences are hidden, making them visible can be a positive step, despite the awkwardness. Being out in the open enables students to locate their peers with LD/ADHD and see that they are not alone. It also makes learning differences seem less mysterious, which in turn can boost students' self-esteem as they recognize that their differences don't mean they are weird or stupid, but part of a valuable and important minority.

Unfortunately, the more visible we become as a community, the greater exposure we have to insensitivity. One of our Eye to Eye chapters recently experienced a challenging incident with a new teacher who used sarcastic humor, especially around learning differences, to try to win his students' approval.

This happens more than you might guess. When people find out you have dyslexia, for example, they assume you flip letters or read backward, and they often make jokes that focus on that misconception. They'll joke with "Tim" and call him "Mit" instead. I remember a teacher who called my friend with ADHD "Bouncing Bobby" because he couldn't sit still.

"Sometimes sarcasm is not good for these kids," one of our ETE supervisors explained. "They don't pick up on it or they don't understand it or they miss those cues. I think you also have to know your kids and when you can be sarcastic. And you really can't use their learning issues as a source of humor unless it's clear that you have that kind of relationship with them."

In addition to his sarcasm, the teacher also singled out the kids with modified testing accommodations in front of the entire class of LD/ADHD and non-LD/ADHD students. The students with LD/ADHD were very upset and asked for help from their supervisor, who told them to talk to their mentors during their next ETE session.

At first, the mentors were very upset. Then they all took a step back and had a great discussion. Together, they decided to write a letter to the teacher explaining why they were so disturbed by his behavior.

When you make light of our learning disabilities in front of the class it makes us feel sad and embarrassed. Also we do not like our other classmates to know about our personal educational styles. We don't want you to be angry with us; we think you're funny and a great teacher. We are not mad at you, but we are mad at our classmates' reactions to your jokes. In the future, please talk to us after class or in the hallway if you're going to talk about our learning styles.

"It was a great moment for the kids and I was proud of them for handling it so well," said the supervisor. "While the incident was hurtful, what they learned from it—that only *they* should determine how people talk about their learning styles—was priceless."

The journey that led these kids from visibility and identity to finally feeling like they were part of a group they could rely on for support and confidence was not a journey we'd want our kids to have, but sometimes it's the painful journeys that are the most empowering.

We may expect kids to be tough on their peers, but it's always a bit shocking when adults exhibit less than thoughtful behavior, especially when those adults are teachers. But this was not the first story I'd heard about an inconsiderate teacher. Teacher bullying is as real as student bullying and we shouldn't assume that all teachers will be understanding when it comes to working with students with LD/ADHD.

Sometimes teachers don't immediately recognize how a particular accommodation can help. While it may be obvious how a ramp helps people in wheelchairs get from point A to point B, the same cannot be said of voice recognition software or a stress ball. It took a while before I was able to articulate why I needed to use a laptop and how it helped me learn. Fortunately, I was surrounded by teachers who were willing to support my different learning style.

For some teachers, there may be a period of adjustment as they learn to work with certain accommodations for the first time. Others may have reactions that demand intervention by school authorities. I've heard of kids being accused of "hiding behind their learning plans" and "using their LD/ADHD as an excuse" far too often. If your child is ever the victim of this kind of attitude, speak to school administrators immediately.

"Some very smart people don't understand learning disabilities and accommodations," says Dr. Koplewicz from the Child Mind Institute. "You have to be able to explain what you really need so your child doesn't have to leave his school, unless you choose that."

It may even be necessary to explain to others that accommodations do not constitute cheating. Because LD/ADHD is invisible, it is much more likely to be misunderstood than other, more visible disabilities are.

Accommodations become even more suspect in testing situations. Unfortunately, some people interpret fairness as meaning we need to teach and test everyone the same way. They don't accept that everyone learns differently. We are sitting on a treasure chest of tools we can use to learn better, but under this idea of fairness, we don't use half of them. What's more, high-stakes testing has turned education on its head; if tests became part of the learning *process* instead of the *result,* we could create a much more equal—and valid—environment in which all learners could thrive.

Until then, parents, students, and their allies and advocates have to do whatever they can—and whatever they're comfortable with—to educate others about different learning styles. Eye to Eye distributes cards that say "I'm a member of the time and a half club" to kids who get extra time on tests. The cards not only make them feel like they belong to a special "club," but they also offer a quick explanation to any detractors. Humor can be used positively, as long as everyone is in on the joke.

Change in any arena usually comes in increments—one step at a time, one accommodation at a time. Technology is making our jobs much, much easier, but the missing piece is social awareness and acceptance. We owe it to our kids and to all the different thinkers of the future to do whatever we can to remove the final obstacles to open and accessible learning for all.

Medication

Medication is an accommodation too, one with its own risks and benefits for kids with ADHD. Determining whether it's a helpful accommodation for your child is a very personal decision, one that should be made with the help and guidance of a qualified health-care professional such as your pediatrician and/or a psychopharmacologist.

Dr. Ned Hallowell's book *Super Parenting for ADHD* describes the moment in 1937 that Dr. Charles Bradley gave hyperactive boys stimulants to help them focus. Until 1937, these boys were judged through a moral framework: they were bad, deviant, unruly, and undisciplined. Dr. Bradley's breakthrough was to treat these behaviors as having a biological, rather than a moral, basis.

He then went on to discover that stimulants helped these boys concentrate. But as Dr. Hallowell points out, stimulants solved one problem—the boys' inability to stay motivated to focus on one activity for long periods of time—while creating a new one. Though the boys were no longer considered *morally* defective, they were now seen as *biologically* defective.

Dr. Hallowell believes we must understand that we identify with our brains differently than we do with any other organ in our body. And because we think of our brains (and their unique challenges) differently than we think of other organs, our reactions to how we treat issues that arise in the brain are also different. It's more personal.

Speaking from a long line of diabetics, I can tell you that no one takes it personally when they are told their pancreas is underperforming and they need to take insulin. However, because our brains are part of our identity, when the assumption is that they need to be "fixed," we must tread more carefully. Instead of judgment, we should exercise thoughtfulness when it comes to ways to help our brains do their jobs better.

The question shouldn't be "Is medication good or bad?" Plenty of research points to the short- and long-term benefits of medication for those with ADHD. Instead, the question should be "Is medication helping me?" If it is (and an experienced doctor is prescribing and monitoring it), use it. If it is not, don't use it.

Medication should be viewed like any other aid used to help folks with LDs get through life: not a fix but a personal accommodation to the world around them, one of many. If students with ADHD embrace a more holistic view of accommodations, it just might empower them to use medication if they find it helpful.

As Hallowell says, "Having ADHD is like having a powerful race car for a brain, but with bicycle brakes. Treating ADHD is like strengthening your brakes—so you start to win races in your life."

We also need to remember that medication is a single tool. It's not enough to give a student Ritalin and then say, "Okay, we're done here." Learning is like building a house—you need a lot of tools. For some of us, Ritalin or Adderall are like hammers. You can build a house without a hammer, but if it's making a critical contribution, why would you throw it out?

Finally, when students are taking medication for ADHD, they need to be aware of how and why it's affecting their learning process. When I was in school, I traipsed to the nurse's office each day for my afternoon dose of Ritalin and had no idea why. I just knew the nurses and teachers thought this pill was supposed to "fix" me and make me better in school.

I still meet students who feel confused and embarrassed about taking the medications that help them get through school. Much of their shame arises from the misguided notion that medication is "wrong"—or that there's a "right" way to cope with ADHD, and medication is not part of that equation.

"To deal with my shame, I used to tell my little brother I'd turn into a werewolf if I didn't take my pill," says Marcus Soutra, ETE's chief operating officer, who was diagnosed with inattentive ADHD and dyslexia in third grade.

"I had a friend with asthma who needed an inhaler and it was completely normalized—but I was hustled down the hall-way for my pill before lunch in a very hush-hush way that sent a clear message: this is somehow shameful or wrong."

Marcus remembers hearing another student screaming that the pill was going to make him different, and soon after he started spitting out his pill because he thought it stunted his creativity and made him "less himself."

"I even thought the pills made me dislike school, though I'm not sure how school would have gone for me had I not been on medication." It wasn't until Marcus reached high school that his parents started talking about his medication as an accommodation.

"I think they finally heard me and realized that if they framed it differently, I'd be more able to benefit from medication rather than fighting it all the time. So my mother began to talk about how I needed my meds for 'game days' when I was having a big test or something, while on days when I didn't need to be as focused—like for field trips—she'd let me skip them."

How we talk about accommodations—especially medication—is almost as important as what the accommodations allow us to accomplish. If kids sense that what they're doing is somehow wrong or shameful, they're naturally going to avoid it. But if they see that using it wisely can be empowering, then they'll get on board.

Students with ADHD often experience several rounds of academic failure before they are diagnosed. For many, medication has been a life-changing accommodation, the difference between success and failure in school. More than students without LD/ADHD, kids with ADHD often need to be praised and celebrated for their learning successes to develop healthy self-esteem and reengage with their schoolwork. If these students start finding success while taking Adderall, then I think we should say, "That's great! You found a tool that's working for you." And then we need to look for more tools.

Finding which tools help us learn takes work, creativity, long-term commitment, and the understanding that there will never be a one-size-fits-all solution for students with ADHD or any other LD. We can also become better listeners. Parents, family members, friends, teachers, and health-care professionals should pay attention to what the Ritalin and Adderall generations have to say about how we succeed with ADHD.

Everyone deserves to learn. Sometimes the best teachers are those who have lived through the experience. That's why ETE has been so successful. It's also why I'm writing this book. As parents, by becoming better listeners—both to your child and to those who have succeeded with learning differences—you too will be able to help.

Accessibility

When ETE started a chapter at Hobart and William Smith Colleges (HWS), I was very excited because the colleges' president was committed to education and service and was the perfect ally for ETE. But it wasn't long before our mentors began to experience trouble.

While they were great at teaching their mentees to be advocates and seek accommodations, they were not accessing accommodations for themselves, even though they knew that's how they would find success in school. In fact, some of the mentors were struggling academically because they hadn't acquired accommodations. Their self-esteem was suffering as a result.

When this story made its way to me, I was shocked, not only because I had such faith in our families and faculty partners, but also because the head of the disability office at HWS had been head of the disability office when I was a student at Brown. She had helped me start ETE and was an advocate for our students.

It turned out that the disability office at HWS was located on the outskirts of campus, next to the counseling office, so that students could maintain a degree of anonymity when requesting accommodations. But the students at HWS were a very empowered bunch, and not only were they not ashamed of their LD/ADHD, they were *proud* of how they learned. In fact, they started ETE's first fraternity/sorority, where students who thought differently could proudly live with and support their fellow LD/ADHD brothers and sisters.

Privacy was not something these kids were looking for. Support was—and even though the support existed, it was so inaccessible as to be useless. The location of the office on the fringes of campus was a logistical challenge to students who already struggled with logistics, and it sent a message that said

"It is on you to make it to the office. The office is not coming to you." This placed the burden on the students rather than recognizing that support should be easy to access, not another hurdle to overcome. Accommodations need to be effective *and* accessible.

Environmental Accommodations

Where we locate the problem is another piece of the accommodations puzzle. Here's a hypothetical example that helps to illustrate this issue.

Every night at six, the Smith family sits down for dinner. Mr. Smith, an avid sports fan, plays the radio to keep up with the latest game scores. The Smiths' two dogs sit under the table and battle over any scraps of food that fall from the table. Lisa, the popular teenager, has a phone that buzzes every five minutes. And the matriarch of the family, Mrs. Smith, asks everyone about their day. By the time it's Joey's turn, he has inevitably zoned out. Mrs. Smith is frustrated that he appears uninterested in the family's daily life, but Joey insists that he just has trouble focusing, a trait apparent in his schoolwork as well.

If we think of it as Joey's *fault*, we can punish or shame him into being a better listener or send him to therapy. We could force him to repeat what everyone has said to make sure he is engaged. These approaches often only mask the problem though and can lead to even greater frustration. But if we think of the environment as at fault, we can take concrete steps to immediately make life easier for Joey—and the whole family. Removing the radio, the pets, and the cell phone could help Joey be a more active participant at dinner.

Clearly, it matters where we locate the problem, though such situations are rarely black and white. In the hypothetical situation with the Smiths, Joey might have also benefited from Adderall or Ritalin. But it is important to look for broader solutions than just "fixing" the student. Similarly, after the students at HWS raised the issue of accessibility, the disability service office moved to the center of campus and they began to get accommodations and find success.

By recognizing that the location of the disability service office was the problem, rather than the students' laziness or indifference, a better solution was found. Moving the office didn't change the students, but it dramatically changed their experience by fixing their environment.

Beyond the classroom, campus, or dinner table, another key environment that plays an integral part in the life of a student with LD/ADHD is his or her bedroom. Bedrooms of kids and teenagers can be chaotically stimulating places: posters of sports stars, bookshelves lined with trophies and photographs, music streaming from multiple sources, buzzing cell phones and pinging IMs. It's hard to imagine how anything gets done in such an environment. Often, nothing does. What's worse, all the other spaces in the house or apartment are sometimes equally noisy and distracting, bad news for kids who need all the help they can get to stay on task.

A friend of mine who struggles with insomnia often talks about sleep hygiene. The first time I heard this phrase, I assumed it had something to do with brushing your teeth. Instead, I learned that my friend makes sure to set herself up properly for a good night's sleep. That means no caffeine after a certain hour, dimmed lights, no LCD screens, and, above all, quiet.

Learning hygiene works very much the same way. We can't expect our children to learn when they are surrounded by chaos. Take the time to set up a quiet and distraction-free study space for your child, even if it means turning off the TV for a while or moving your toddler into another room. This may be easier said than done, especially when space is limited, and it's not something most kids request—often, they don't even realize they need it. But it's crucial to ensure proper study environments exist somewhere in a home for children to learn without distraction.

Let's Not Wait for the Future

As I've already mentioned, there is an element of paradox in our understanding of LD/ADHD. While neuroimaging technology has shown that LD/ADHD brains are different from non-LD/ADHD brains, we also know that teaching methods and environmental factors play a huge role in whether or not people with LD/ADHD are successful academically. As our understanding of LD/ADHD brains improves, so does our ability to teach those different brains.

Science and technology also help create better learning environments. My ancient laptop is a prime example; once a unique accommodation, now many students, LD/ADHD and non-LD/ADHD alike, depend on laptops and tablets to learn better. In fact, many schools and universities expect or even require the use of tablets as a teaching aid. One day, other accommodations such as voice-recognition software may become as accepted and maybe as common as computers— and will likely be overshadowed by even greater advances.

Strong memorization skills may become less critical as students are allowed to rely more on technology and less on memory to recall information that can be quickly and easily accessed by all students. Older generations will have to accept that change rather than rail against it. The fact that the SAT and ACT now allow calculators is just one more indication that we are beginning to accept the use of helpful technology by *all* students, not just those with learning disabilities.

What I'm hoping to convey in this chapter, however, is that we must still do whatever we can to help children learn better *now*. If that means locating technology to assist, then let's do it. If it means using alternative teaching methods, let that be a piece of the solution as well. It's important to question the primacy of certain teaching methods and approaches.

Although we all are familiar with the crippling limitations on school budgets and resources, many of the solutions that already exist are neither expensive nor resource-depleting. They're just different. And sometimes change is hard. As a parent of a child with a learning difference, you are part of the team that can make a difference in how everyone learns. In the next chapter, we'll look at ways to make sure your child is taking full advantage of those changes and working smarter.

Chapter 6

WORK SMARTER

One reason I have confidence in my writing
is I have confidence in my stamina.

—John Irving, author, dyslexic

Many kids with LD/ADHD want nothing more than to excel. They simply don't know *how*. Schools assume that everyone knows how to work hard and that if you do, success will follow.

Unfortunately, we all know this is not always the case. As parents, you may need to help your child discover what it means to work *smarter*—by knowing how her brain works and using her accommodations—to bring her closer to her goals.

Take the Chairlift When You Can

When I decided to get my master's in education, I chose Columbia's dis/Abilities Studies Program for a variety of reasons, not the least of which was the defiant way they spelled *dis/Ability*. My hope was to find a group of like-minded people interested in exploring the state of education; specifically, what was disenfranchising smart students in our schools at an alarming rate.

With that lofty goal in mind, I set off for northern Manhattan every morning from my Brooklyn apartment. It was a long train ride, and I made sure to use the time wisely, working on reading assignments and doing my best to stay ahead of my classes. The good news was that I no longer faced a stream of distractions as I had in college—no late-night pizza parties, no noisy friends stumbling into my room to pull me away from the reading that took me twice as long to finish anyway.

As with most schools of higher learning, Columbia did things in a very specific—and very traditional—way. Despite the fact that I was in a program progressively titled dis/Ability Studies, in order to pass my classes, I was still expected to read, write papers, and take tests. Although I had mastered *that* way, I knew it wasn't the *best* way for me to learn because it took so much extra effort. It didn't actually deepen my learning.

It was as if I was at a great ski resort whose tradition maintained that skiers *walked* up the hill, and everyone obliged. I wanted to take a chairlift. Walking would have been harder, not smarter, because the goal was skiing, not walking up the hill. At Columbia, my goal was to learn, not to trudge up a hill to get to learn. I loved learning and knew I could do it the hard way—by walking up the hill—or the better way, by taking the chairlift. For me, that meant learning interactively with teachers who would challenge and engage me.

One reason I chose Columbia was that the authors of the textbooks we used in the classroom were actually on the faculty. As much as I could, I tried to enroll in classes taught by teachers I'd have face-to-face access to. I ignored "tradition" and the read/study/write paradigm and jumped on the chairlift as much as possible.

To me, the most compelling professor at Columbia—perhaps the single biggest draw to me as a student—was a woman named Maxine Greene. I'd been reading her work since I was eighteen and couldn't wait to study under her. Unfortunately, there were no classes with her available to me; because she was elderly, she was only teaching students further along in their studies.

Since I was used to going around obstacles rather than simply accepting them, my different-thinking brain kicked in and realized I could reach out to her directly rather than just accept the status quo. Even though I didn't have her e-mail, I knew that all Columbia professors' e-mail followed the same pattern, so I crafted a heartfelt appeal to Professor Greene and sent it into the ether.

I didn't ask for much—I just wanted to take her to lunch—and I made certain to let her know that I was very familiar with her work and that it directly tied into the national art-based mentoring program I was launching. One of her big arguments is that art often functions as a form of democracy and can be both freeing and empowering. I had already witnessed this in Eye to Eye and couldn't wait to discuss it with her over pie and coffee.

Well, one lunch turned into dozens, as we proceeded to meet weekly for the two years I was at Columbia. At the end of our time together, which I managed to arrange as an independent study project, I could have just written a paper, but instead I created a video project about how ETE fit in with Professor Greene's philosophy. The project took far longer than writing a paper would have, but this time, working harder was also smarter, as the process of making the video taught me far more than I would have learned writing a paper.

It also reinforced my formula for learning that I had discovered in college:

ME + BOOKS = OK
ME + PEOPLE = BETTER

Grad school was the first time I got a 4.0. But for the first time in my academic career, I never once thought about my grades. Because I was studying what I loved and doing it on my terms, I excelled. Most people would excel in these conditions.

The problem is, obviously, that these conditions—when passion is strong, obstacles limited, and motivation high—are usually missing or in short supply in most academic environments, especially in grammar and middle schools. That's why ETE has had such a huge impact on the populations it has touched. We help kids find their passion, teach them how to minimize obstacles (or overcome them completely), and, through the example of our mentors, provide them with motivation to work harder and smarter—often for the first time in their young lives.

As parents, the question is how to cultivate these conditions in your child's academic career. How to raise passionate, engaged kids? How to help remove impediments to their learning style? How to motivate them to *work*?

The answers, as I've begun to outline in this book, begin with identifying their strengths and weaknesses, uncovering how they learn best, and seeking the right accommodations for their learning style. But kids—and even some adults—also need to learn *how* to work, both in the classroom and beyond. For me, that lesson crystallized after I graduated and began working.

Learning How to Work

When I applied to be a Brown University admissions officer shortly after I graduated, the job application process mirrored the way I like to think: interpersonally and hands-on. Brown gave me the files of four students who had either been accepted or rejected. I had to review their applications and discuss the strength of each with my fellow admissions officers. I loved that I would be judged on how well I actually did the job, not on how well I argued I'd be able to do it.

Each file was more interesting than the previous and each represented great potential. I was hooked. I immediately saw that this job would give me a lens into students' individual lives, as well as a sense of the schools they attended and what education was like for them. While my Brown majors in education and psychology had helped me develop a fine theoretical perspective on education in America and my student teaching had given me a very specific slice of life in the classroom, this job would give me the best of both worlds.

I walked into my interview a proud person with ADHD and dyslexia. After I was done sharing my thoughts on the applicants, I went on to talk about my work in ETE. I spoke of my experiences with ADHD and dyslexia and when they asked how quickly I could read, I was honest. Since the job entailed reading two thousand student applications a year, my supervisors wondered if I might need some kind of accommodations. I told them that I had read books and kept up with my peers at Brown, which seemed to dispel their concerns. I got the job and was chosen to be the office's disability liaison as well, in charge of reading all student files that made any reference to disability.

I was thrilled I was going to be able to look out for my people.

Let me pause and openly admit that selecting a job where my primary function five months out of the year was to read, a weakness of mine that came with full professional certification, was perhaps not the wisest choice. But my decoding skills were still serving me well and though I might have been a slower reader than some of my fellow admissions officers, I also knew I could outwork them. Work had become a skill as much as a value.

While my dyslexia was central in my mind going into the position, I somehow managed to forget about my ADHD. It did not forget about me.

Most of the admissions officers had private offices that were tucked into the nooks and crannies of the two-hundred-year-old admissions office. As the youngest and least experienced staffer, I shared an office with a gregarious young woman named Jackie, who always finished reading her two dozen files by lunchtime, when I'd usually be about halfway through my third file.

She clearly learned and processed information by speaking and read her files out loud, conjuring the spirit of each applicant so she could have a mock interview. I found this deeply amusing and immensely distracting. The afternoon would include a carousel of visitors due to Jackie's popularity.

If this was not enough of an ADHD nightmare, visiting students created a constant rumble on the other side of our office door. Inevitably, just when I was getting somewhere, my boss would call me into an unscheduled meeting and whatever application I was in the middle of would require a full reread.

No amount of Adderall, noise-canceling headphones, or Do Not Disturb signs would have produced an environment that enabled me to focus on reading two dozen student applications a day for five months straight. After a few days of this chaos, I knew I needed to ask for help.

I did not want to call attention to the problems I was facing with my job; I just wanted to get back on track and consider some ideas for altering my working environment. I prepared to approach my boss the same way I had approached every other authority figure before her: first with kindness (Will you help me?) and then with firmness (The Americans with Disabilities Act says you *have* to help me!).

My supervisor welcomed me into her office but before I could begin, she said, "David, do you know you are more than a hundred files behind your quota?" I knew that our work was tracked, but I had no idea how closely.

"Yes," I meekly replied.

"I'm concerned that the way you are going about the work is not, well . . . working?" I assumed she was referring to my dyslexia but didn't want to use the word *reading* so she used *work* instead. I knew this routine. In our politically correct world, she didn't know how to talk about the problem for fear of insulting me or, worse, appearing to discriminate. But the real problem was that she thought my issue was the reading, while it was actually the distraction-filled office. I carefully tried to clarify.

"You know when you go out to dinner with a friend and

want to have a serious conversation, but the restaurant seats you by the kitchen? You feel awkward but you ask the waiter if there is a quieter table, maybe something in the back or in a corner?" I could tell by the look on her face that she had no idea what I was talking about, but she told me to continue.

"I am reading my files right next to the kitchen." As the words came out of my mouth, I realized I had not used the best metaphor. Confirming this, she said exactly what she had been so hesitant to say before.

"What does this have to do with your dyslexia?"

I began to laugh, in part because I knew she had just walked into a new world—a dis/ABILITY world—and I was her welcoming committee. I rebooted and tried again.

"When I applied for this job, I spoke openly about my dyslexia and explained that while reading the files might take me longer, I was willing to put in the extra hours, or the equivalent of the extra time on tests I received while a student here at Brown. What we did not discuss was my ADHD."

She waited for me to continue.

"You see, it's really not a *deficit* in attention, it's a *surplus* of attention. I have no blinders; it all streams in and my office is like the Mississippi River."

"So what should we do?" she asked, looking to me to lead the way. "I need you to catch up."

"Can I start reading from home? I'll sign whatever's necessary to take responsibility for anything that might happen to the files once they leave the office. I promise to catch up and stay on track. I just need to be in an environment I can control a bit more."

Her answer was one I'd heard before.

"If we do this for you, then we have to do this for everyone."

I responded exactly as I had in my testing days.

"I think that's a *great* idea!"

At first, she asked me just to "try harder." I explained how that game had already played its course with me unsuccessfully in grade school. More than ten years later, it still didn't help me.

As I got further behind, my supervisor relented and, yes, everyone was permitted to take their files home to read. It was a calculated risk but she needed the job done. Along with the rest of my admissions officers, we did just that. We got the job done.

At the end of the day, that is what all individuals with LD/ADHD want: to get the job done, whether it's on a school project or one at the office. As different thinkers, we have to work hard at almost everything we do. Part of the reason for that is to compensate for problematic learning environments. But sometimes obstacles can teach us valuable lessons.

Compensatory Mechanisms

Without even knowing it, different thinkers begin to develop what are called *compensatory mechanisms* as soon as they hit a snag. I'm not talking about taking a trip to the restroom when there's a chance they might have to read aloud in class. Instead, I'm referring to the things every human does to make up for a weakness or missing skill set.

Let's say your car has a blind spot on the right-hand rear side. Chances are you can find a way around this blind spot, either by turning your head to look behind you or using the passenger-side mirror more thoughtfully. In effect, you are compensating for the design of your car. It's still a great car—heck, maybe it's even a Ferrari—but it isn't perfect. The important thing is to know its limitations and learn how to work around them so that it can reach its peak performance safely.

The same idea works with your brain. Some of our brains have a hard time reading pages with a lot of text. To help it out, perhaps we cover up all but two or three lines of text at a time so that our brain isn't overwhelmed. Does that mean our brains are defective? Of course not. In fact, it might make us really good at seeing the big picture or the broader scope of ideas. While some people are better able to focus on details, or the micro level of things, others excel at seeing the macro version. Some academic subjects even differentiate between these two approaches—economics, for example, has macro and micro fields. You can bet that people are drawn to study whichever type comes more easily to them.

Other kinds of compensatory mechanisms are quite simple. To dispel ADHD energy, some kids jiggle their legs or chew gum. If you know that fidgeting helps your child focus, then you can seek appropriate accommodations, perhaps by suggesting he use a stress ball or by getting permission for him to chew gum quietly during tests.

Many of these tricks are simply ways to modify unfriendly learning environments, and they can be a boon to different thinkers, even if it sometimes feels like we have to work harder to achieve the same results as our peers. But another reason for why we must sometimes work so hard has to do with perception. A frustrating aspect of being learning disabled is that expectations for us are often lower.

Low Expectations and the LD Student

When people know someone has LD/ADHD, they often lower the bar for what they think that person can achieve. This is just plain wrong and something we all need to try to change. When we first started ETE, I did my best to combat low expectations by meeting them head-on and working smarter.

I distinctly remember the day I went with a handful of future ETE mentors to get the supervising dean's official sign-off to start ETE. Dean M's office was in the stately redbrick building known as University Hall, which had housed far more significant conversations than the one we were about to have. However, in our minds, this was the most important conversation this building would have for the foreseeable future. We figured we were about to plant the seeds for a movement to change education, starting with a group of kids just like us. We were also going to turn the entire approach to LD/ADHD on its head by including folks who thought differently in the process. Very simply, we thought we were going to make history.

And we were fifteen minutes late.

Dean M was a legend in the field of LD/ADHD—from our vantage point, the pope of LD/ADHD. His blessing would mean we could go forward with our idea; his rejection, the end of the road. I had a full eight inches on him, but I was nervous to the bone. He had a round benevolent face and seemed like the kind of person who would always take the side of the underdog. I just knew we had to make him *our guy*.

When we arrived, he had no idea why we were there. First, I apologized for being late. Then I continued.

"When school was difficult for me as a kid, my parents tried to motivate me by saying, 'Tom Cruise is dyslexic and look at him!' While I was a huge fan, I couldn't understand how someone who didn't go to college was supposed to help me." I continued by explaining how as Brown students with LD/ADHD, we were uniquely suited to be mentors for young students with LD. Then each of my peers enthusiastically shared similar stories.

Judging by the look on Dean M's face, he was clearly weighing the possibility of our idea's success *and* failure.

"You have something wonderful here. In fact, in my decades in the field, I have never heard such an interesting and generous initiative. But let's think about this for a minute. We have a whole office designed to help you find success here at Brown. Don't get me wrong, we know you are smart—that's why you are here—but the very challenges you face in school are going to be the limitations you face as mentors. I mean, you were all fifteen minutes late." He paused for impact. "Maybe we should leave this to the professionals."

After we apologized again for being late, he said he would think about our proposal.

That night, I lay in my dorm room bed, my feet hanging off the edge. I lamented how my lanky six-foot-two frame did not quite fit on the one-size-fits-all twin bed. *Nothing ever fits,* I thought to myself. *My brain doesn't fit in school and my body doesn't fit in this bed.* I then decided to do something I never had done without significant parental prodding. I wrote a thank-you e-mail.

Dear Dean M,

Thank you so much for taking the time to meet with us today. Eye to Eye is something we believe could help young students finally see a road map for their success and help our teachers and parents better understand and support their kids. Furthermore, we think we can learn from this as well, and perhaps help rewrite our own histories, doing for these students what we wish had been done for us. Your support would

mean everything to us and who knows, might change
the world forever . . .

Thanks for your consideration,
Your future Eye to Eye mentors

P.S. Sorry again for being late. It won't happen again,
to you, or anyone, ever.

In another moment of uncharacteristic self-awareness, I went down the hall and asked a cute girl I knew was an English major to proofread the note. I then pressed send. The postscript sat with me.

The next day, Dean M signed off on the program. A week later, the head of the Swearer Center for Public Service backed us and so did the head of the Brown Education Department. Finally, but most important, the head of the Special Education Program at Fox Point Elementary invited us to meet her students.

I could easily have just given up when Dean M told us to "leave this to the professionals." But I knew that by taking that extra step and making my case to him, at least I would have done everything I could to launch my dream.

Eye to Eye was born through faith and by individuals who viewed me and my mentors through a lens of potential. Although these amazing people did not judge us by our limitations, the cautionary words of Dean M stuck. He chose to see beyond our perceived limitations, but I understood this was the exception and not the rule. It's not fair that LD/ADHDers face so many inaccurate assumptions, but if we work together, we can try to dispel the myths around LD/ADHD.

Exceeding Expectations

Even the people who love us and support us don't always believe we can get past our limitations. The only way we are going to gain that acceptance is by raising the bar. Yes, ADHD sometimes makes us disorganized and late. That means we have to be proactive and use accommodations to confront our challenges. Yes, reading and spelling are tough for us; that means we always need to use a spell-checker and leave extra time for rereading things that are important. The more important the meeting or paper, the more on top of our game we have to be.

A recent book looks at the path of so-called superachievers to distill what enables people to reach their goals. In addition to being able to constantly evaluate their progress and make corrections to their path, successful people were also found to be incredibly patient and to surround themselves with people who supported them. As we learned in chapter 4, relying on metacognition is an important element in the success of any different thinker. In later chapters, we'll learn how essential allies and advocates are for LD/ADHD success.

But having goals—stepping up to and even exceeding

expectations—can enable different thinkers to achieve more than anyone thought they could.

As Camille Sweeney and Josh Gosfield wrote in their column "Secret Ingredient for Success," in the *New York Times:*

> . . . *what we learned from conversation with high achievers is that challenging our assumptions, objectives, at times even our goals, may sometimes push us further than we thought possible.*

Although this may help explain the success of superachievers, there's nothing to keep the rest of us from benefiting from it as well.

First, sometimes hard work *doesn't* result in the outcome you want. But with the right perspective, this kind of failure can be a great opportunity. For one, it's good to learn what you're *not* good at. And if you haven't tried your hardest, you can't be sure whether your failure is the result of not trying or just not being skilled at something. Knowing your strengths and weaknesses is essential for all of us, but especially for those of us with LD/ADHD. Since it's often our responsibility to reshape our learning environments to better suit our brains, it helps to know in advance what we're good at and what we need help with. And test results don't always tell us that; failure does.

In *Jonathan Livingston Seagull,* Richard Bach tells the

story of an unusual bird who chooses to defy his flock by seeking more from life than fish scraps. His persistence and intense desire to learn new things lead him to an exceptional life, one in which every problem or failure is an opportunity in disguise. This may be one of the many reasons that so many successful entrepreneurs are LD/ADHD. In fact, more than a third of the entrepreneurs surveyed in a 2007 study by Julie Logan of the Cass Business School in London said they were dyslexic. In order to succeed in the tough world of business, not only do they have to be willing to fail, but they also need to learn from their mistakes.

Speaking of flying, two very successful airline CEOs— Virgin Atlantic's Richard Branson and Jet Blue's David Neeleman both have learning issues. Branson admits that for a long time he didn't know the difference between net and gross profits. One of his board members finally caught on to his charade and gave him a mnemonic device, or a clever aid to help him remember.

"Pretend you're fishing," his friend told him. "Net is all the fish in your net at the end of the year. Gross is that plus everything that got away."

Creative and unique problem-solving skills are among the many strengths of different thinkers and often enable them to overcome obstacles that would defeat less resilient folks. It's something I keep in mind when I work with ETE's volunteers, who are always gunning to exceed expectations that others set for them.

"We want the world to expect greatness from us, but for that to happen, we have to demonstrate greatness ourselves," says ETE's COO Marcus Soutra.

We must also live our values.

For the past ten years we've held a national training conference for ETE's core LD/ADHD leaders, who are all between ages sixteen and twenty-two. We spend five days teaching them how to lead by example in their respective communities. While they are incredibly diverse in experiences, religion, culture, socioeconomic background, race, gender, and sexual orientation, they are united by their different thinking and a commitment to be the change the world needs so desperately. We've lovingly referred to it as LDpalooza.

This is what I tell our trainees:

There is no underage drinking or drug use.

Why? Because that is what society expects and we can't afford to feed into that stereotype.

We expect you to be on time.

Why? Because everyone else expects us to be late.

We invest in you!

Why? Because you are the professionals on LD/ADHD.

We trust you to lead your communities when you get back home.

Why? Because you are symbols of success.

Never once have I had to send anyone home early. What's more, every single attendee has gone on to become an exemplary leader. I would trust each and every one of our mentors to care for my children.

By exceeding expectations, we smooth the road for those who follow.

Now let's talk about some of the more quotidian kinds of work we need to do as different thinkers. I just threw something into that last sentence that is emblematic of a kind of challenge *all* students face, but for those with LD/ADHD, it's important not to miss. I used what I call a "ten-dollar word"—*quotidian*. Some students know what it means, some don't. But how many kids who don't know would bother to look it up? And how many would miss it completely?

Simple challenges such as unknown vocabulary words arise every day. But only the most conscientious and ambitious students bother to (1) notice and (2) step up to the challenge. Students with LD/ADHD need to do both, perhaps even more so than their non-LD/ADHD peers. It goes back to that idea of exceeding expectations with every opportunity that comes along.

We're like the short kids on the basketball team—we have to be great shots, quick and strategic. Floating along on our height just isn't an option. We have to overcompensate for our "weaknesses" so that we can compete with the tall people. Yet remember: the basketball court is one of the few places where being short is a legitimate weakness. In other situations, shortness is an asset (see: jockeys).

Similarly, LD/ADHD can be a tremendous asset. And

a "difference" is only a difference on certain courts with specific rules. A short person might excel at gymnastics or wrestling, and someone with LD/ADHD might excel in a hands-on classroom like one involving circuitry and technology. The environment and the rules of that environment—not so-called intelligence or IQ—predict success.

The best answers are often stumbled on, just as mine were. But asking the right questions is an essential first step. Too many parents just want their kids to work harder, when harder, as I learned, is not always better. Smarter is always better. Working harder is what happens when passion kicks in. I worked both harder *and* smarter in grad school because I was following my passion, and all my assignments had great relevance to my life.

Relevance is a tough thing to find in grammar school. But we can still try to help our kids by improving their learning environments and exposing them to inspiring and motivating ideas, people and goals. All it takes is one spark to start a fire if the kindling is ready. So set down the kindling and throw a few sparks in the right direction. Then step back and watch it catch fire.

Chapter 7

FIND YOUR ALLIES

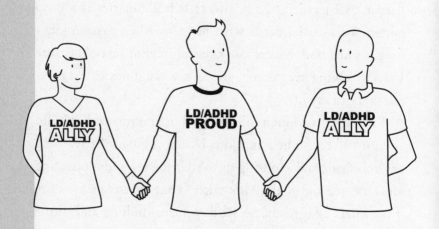

I had a grandmother . . .
who was telling me I was special. . . .
She just said, "You're going to find
your way through this. Think big, be big."
—Brian Grazer, film and television producer, dyslexic

Even the most determined kids can't do it all on their own, no matter how confident and resilient they are. They need a network of supportive allies to serve as a safety net one day, and maybe a cheerleading section the next. That network begins at home with you.

It All Starts at Home

I don't have vivid memories of the report cards I brought home in sealed manila envelopes for my parents. The results were rarely surprising (when you don't finish most of the test, you have a pretty good sense you are not passing), so perhaps that's why my grades were rarely discussed.

However, after attending Schenck, my family gained a renewed faith in my abilities. And with the help of my laptop, customized reading techniques, audio books, and a number of other accommodations and tools, I was acing Galloway—in everything but science. In tenth grade, we switched to a new biology textbook that lacked an audio version. My decoding skills were good, but every other word in biology is brand-new, so getting through the text took twice as long as my usual sluggish speed. When my report card came home that semester, the dinner table was where we hashed it out.

Even before that report card appeared, my dad and I chose the dinner table to discuss our differences, though the fodder was usually something in the news, sports, or politics. We even fought about the definitions of words—my father has an amazing vocabulary and loves to show off. It is pretty common for teens to fight with their parents and especially common for those whose are deeply similar, as I am with my ADHD dad.

So when my report card showed up, the first to reflect my new struggles in science, I mentally put on my armor. The man across the table dealt with his ADHD very differently than I did. His solution to everything was to "try harder," which I had already learned didn't work for me. My understanding and acceptance of my LD/ADHD had taught me how to use accommodations to go around obstacles, rather than through them, as my father often did. But he didn't have dyslexia—in fact, he was a big reader. His ADHD just kept him from finishing the books he started.

Furthermore, my father had invested more money in my

education than we spent on any other single expense in our family. An investment like that warranted results. As my dad opened the report card, I braced myself. He looked through the grades and his eyes fell upon my C-.

"So what happened here in science?"

"Don't you mean what happened with all my other classes? What about my top marks in English, history, math . . . ?"

"Yes, they are noted," he said very steadily. "But what's the story with science?"

Utilizing the same strategy I learned in grade school when things started looking bleak, I quickly retreated and locked myself in my room. Eventually, my mother knocked on my door with my untouched dinner and left without saying a word. When I heard my parents start to argue a few minutes later, I blocked it out.

An hour passed and another light knock rapped on my door. I thought it was my mother; when my father's shadow came over me, I froze.

"What are you working on?" He tried to sound neutral, but I knew he was constructing an argument. "Have you started science yet?"

"Nope."

My father's father was a florist who ran a small shop called Flink's Flowers in LaGrange, Georgia. My grandfather was not around to help my dad with school, but that wasn't unusual back then. My dad just worked really hard, which he no doubt learned from his father. So when he came to my room, I expected some strong words about the importance of pushing through.

Instead, he said, "Can I help?"

As a teenager, I had not quite caught on that we were writing a new script, so I responded with attitude.

"You want to *help*?" I asked, incredulous. "You *really* want to help? Why don't you read it to me?"

I think I might have even thrown in an "old man" at the end of the sentence just to add some extra dynamite to the mix. Then life took a new course. My father picked up the book and left the room. Two seconds later, he came back to ask what chapter I was on.

"The class is on chapter four, but I still haven't finished reading chapter one."

I soon heard a muffled voice through the paper-thin walls of our house. My father was reading the text, and I quickly realized that he must be taping himself. Since my dad is ADHD and not dyslexic, he had no trouble reading as long as he could pace the floors. He returned later that evening and put both the book and the tape recorder on my desk.

He had been a radio announcer in college, so his beautiful speaking voice transformed the text from inedible symbols to a protein shake of sound. I inhaled the content, hungry to finally understand what had been going on in class. Over time, the microtapes began to pile up so high I had to create a special storage system to keep them all straight. Like magic, my grades started to go up.

Sometimes your best accommodation is an ally.

If I ever wondered who had my back or needed someone to believe in me, I need look no further than the skyscraper of tapes with my father's voice revealing the miracles of science and, even more important, how much he loved and believed in me. Good grades were simply a by-product. To this day, the second drawer on the left of my childhood desk contains an audio collection of Miller and Levine's *Biology*. I now keep one tape with me wherever I go. Although I no longer need its content, the support it symbolizes reminds me that no challenge is too great, especially with great allies.

Allies Are Everywhere

Some of the greatest allies in my life were people I didn't even know were my allies. Kids are drawn to people who support them; that support can come in surprising ways. In fourth grade, I was spending more and more time in the hall outside my classroom as payment for impulsive interruptions, lost homework assignments, intercepted cheating, or as an accommodation meant to individualize my education but which only made me feel singled out and isolated.

Towering over us little kids in his sky blue custodial uniform, Jim walked the halls of my school with a ready smile, reserving his biggest smiles for those who needed them most.

One day, my mother overheard the assistant principal, Dr. S, telling Jim, "We pay you to clean, and we pay them [the teachers] to teach. Let's let everyone do what they do best." I remember the *how-dare-she* look on my mother's face as she recounted the story. After Dr. S's comments, Jim handed out his smiles to students more cautiously. A line had been drawn and he dared not cross it.

In a way, both Jim and I had been singled out and isolated. Yet Jim had worked at my school for a very long time, and he had seen two other assistant principals come and go. I suspect he knew he would outlast Dr. S as well, though his job was still on the line, which made his willingness to buoy my spirit all the more heroic.

The two of us continued to exchange smiles as part of his end-of-the-day sweep, which often coincided with my daily excommunication from class. I'd hear him coming around the corner and by the time he made the turn, I was already up on my feet, ready to offer my best high five (a rather low five for the six-foot giant). Still, Jim and I dared not speak. However we communed, somehow I felt he understood me, perhaps better than anyone else in my life at that time.

Months into my hallway ritual with Jim, something got the better of him and he asked why I was always in the hallway.

"Are you making sure I do my job?" he inquired with a smile.

At first, I was taken aback. I thought I was going to have to defend why I was outside and I did not have a very good answer. When I realized he was joking, I replied, "Yup, keep up the good work, Jim!"

"That's not fair. You know my name, but I don't know yours." I told him my name and he silently moved along. That was the end of our first real conversation, but it was the best day I'd had in school for a long time.

Two sentences at a time, we came to know each other better and I began to feel like someone finally understood me. He would try to guess what brought me to his hallway. One day, he came down the hall and instead of our usual two-sentence exchange, he reached into a hidden pocket of his uniform and pulled out a small chess set. Either Jim was very bad at the game or he let me win a lot. Regardless, it was a gift and a very empowering one at that.

I will never know why Jim chose to be a custodian in my school. I won't know why he offered smiles to kids who needed them the most even if it risked his job. And I won't know if he had been a kid like me who sat outside his classroom day in and day out. What I do know is Jim was my salvation. In fourth grade, if not for Jim, his smiles, and his chess set, I would have given up.

Knowing exactly what a child needs and when is a difficult skill to master. Somehow Jim could see I was suffering and managed to connect with me in a way that was unlike attempts by any other adult in my life.

Only one other person ever came close, and that was my uncle David.

In Jewish tradition, you are not supposed to be named after someone living, so my uncle and I were both named after my grandfather's father, who lost his life in the concentration camps. However, I knew that secretly I was named after Uncle David. He was all the things a cool uncle should be: athletic, a classic sports car owner, and my unconditional ally. While Jim saved me at my Jewish day school, Uncle David came to my rescue during my horrible year at the college prep school.

When the bright yellow Bluebird bus would pull in from its journey, my uncle would be there, sitting on the hood of his '68 GTO ready to whisk me away. I would feel the powerful engine of the car as the wind blew, and for a brief time, I'd enjoy complete escape. Other days, we'd toss a Frisbee back and forth and he'd tell me how he survived being bullied. "You can't reason with unreasonable people," he'd say, and I would hold this in my heart for strength.

We shared more than our name and love of Frisbee; we shared a lens into the hidden world of disability, though his journey had been much deeper and more painful than mine. On May 8, 1992, an eighteen-wheel tractor trailer rammed his car, killing his wife and causing my uncle to have a traumatic brain injury.

As he mourned the loss of his wife, he also had to come to grips with the challenges of having a disability. Though you could never guess it when you saw him sitting on the hood of his GTO, he spent years relearning how to speak, walk, and even swallow. The repercussions of what became an invisible disability were still vast as he continued to teach his brain tasks it once knew well. Sometimes, he had to alter the outside world to enable his brain to function, something I had learned to do as well. As we tossed the Frisbee or zoomed down country roads, we spoke openly about how to use accommodations to succeed at everyday tasks.

Both Jim and my uncle David provided me with the kind of support no parent or teacher could. Perhaps their unique perspectives on difference enabled them to connect with me in a way others couldn't. That kind of empathy is part of what led me to help start Eye to Eye and is also why the program has been so successful.

Peer Allies

Our ETE mentors are uniquely positioned to understand and identify with many of the struggles our young mentees face because they have been through the same struggles themselves. From using their fists to differentiate between lower-case "b"s and "d"s (put your fists together and your thumbs up and press: you have a "d" on your right hand, and a "b" on your left) to wearing hair bands on their wrists to tell right from left, our mentors have a whole host of tricks and insights and want to share that knowledge with their mentees.

We have also mastered the sleight of hand when it comes to getting kids to do something they might not normally do, like open up about their LD/ADHD. By diverting their attention with a supercool art project, we can then pepper the session with all kinds of questions and conversations about what it means to be LD/ADHD and how to feel more empowered.

Rarely do our mentees realize that our volunteers are the magicians of the mentoring world. Before they even know it, the mentees have shared stories and struggles for the first time in their lives. That sharing builds the bridge from their little island of one to a whole community of different thinkers, where resources and support flourishes and everyone can learn freely and openly.

Finding allies with shared experience is invaluable to *any* kid, not just those with LD/ADHD. Often, allies are simply the conduit for kids to realize their own greatness, facilitators rather than teachers or coaches. Eye to Eye doesn't teach kids anything academic; all our work is done through art projects, specially crafted to help kids discover things about themselves no other process—traditional classroom activities, therapy, tutoring—has enabled them to find. The confidence kids access in our program spills over into the rest of their lives—in schoolwork, in relationships with others, and in their aspirations for themselves.

Perhaps the most important by-product of our work is that kids raise expectations for themselves and what they can achieve, not just because they work with older students who are well on their way to greatness, but because for the first time in the lives, they *feel good* about who they are and what they can accomplish. Sometimes that starts with a superhero cape or the transformation of a lunch box into a personal talisman.

A few years ago, I saw great teamwork in action at one of our local ETE chapters.

Spunky and fun, a quintessential California girl, even though she was a student at Vassar College in chilly upstate New York, Susie K carried with her the warmth of the California sun everywhere she went: you want her as your mentor. When I met with her after the ETE training on her campus, she enthusiastically asked me rapid-fire questions. *How can I be the best mentor possible for my student? What if I don't have anything to advise my student on? What will I do if I can't get them to open up to me?*

I told her to rely on her gut and teach what she knew. I could see she had an old soul and that even though we had only finished the first day of training, she could have walked into the life of almost any kid and made a difference.

When I next visited, Susie and her mentee had been working together for months. An eighth grader, Jacob was a string bean of a teenager, about the same height as Susie. From a distance, you might not be able to tell the mentor from the mentee. However, on closer inspection, Jacob's body language told it all: frustration sealed into the body of a boy. Though he had plenty to say, he rarely said much at all and when he did, it was quietly.

Before introducing myself to Jacob, I asked the ETE liaison at Jacob's school about Jacob's story. She had a sixth sense about kids and could read them like tea leaves. More like a prediction than an observation, she told me, "Jacob is very smart, but no one in his world believes this, even him. Susie sees his brilliance."

I was struck by the maturity Susie displayed with her mentee, engaging with Jacob in what seemed like a well-choreographed dance. They had become of one mind and had clearly bonded. I asked about the project they were working on. Jacob gave Susie a glance that seemed to say *Can we trust this guy?* Susie, aware that it was the same project we had covered in our training, played along.

"Jacob, why don't we let David in on what we're doing? After all, he is one of us." She said this with a gentle smile that showed me their intense trust. It was clear Susie made sure no one threatening entered Jacob's world, at least not on her watch.

Jacob remained focused on his project. In short sentences, he explained that the box in front of him was a metaphor for himself. The inside of the box represented how he felt in school and the exterior of the box showed how he wished the outside world actually saw him. I was impressed at how succinctly he had summed up a project that had taken me days to express in our curriculum. Their supervisor was right: smart kid.

I left the pair and worked my way around the room, but I couldn't stop looking back at Jacob. There was something extremely familiar about him, perhaps because he reminded me of myself at his age.

Finally, as the art projects were being brought to a close, I floated back to Jacob and Susie and saw that Jacob was about to superglue his box shut permanently.

"Can I ask why you're doing that, Jacob?"

"What's inside is for Susie and me to know. That's it."

As he finished affixing the lid, forever sealed, I noticed the outside of the box for the first time. Simply and elegantly, Jacob had cut out letters from a magazine and written *JACOB*. Next to that, he wrote: *Smarter than you think he is.*

The projects were to be put on display for teachers and peers to appreciate the creativity and effort. Jacob had decided to use this opportunity to rebrand himself, if you will. With Susie's help, he learned he was smart. Now he wanted to make sure the rest of the world knew it too.

Eye to Eye art projects serve many different purposes. On the most basic level, they help the mentor and mentee build a relationship and have a conversation. We put their art on display as much to celebrate these relationships as to celebrate the discoveries the students have made while doing the projects. While many students with LD/ADHD do show an innate predilection for art, we aren't teaching art as much as doing art for art's sake.

Jacob's project was a shining example of what is possible when we allow students to be creative and dream. Through his work with Susie, Jacob not only found a way to believe he was smart, but he also was able to share this new belief with the rest of the world. The idea of "smart" is probably the hardest thing to convey to a kid with LD/ADHD. Even with accommodations and support, every kid must go through an often exceptionally challenging obstacle course in order to understand that kids with LD/ADHD might show their smarts differently from the other 80 percent of their peers.

Mentoring

Having an older role model, especially one who is also LD/ADHD and knows the ropes, can be an invaluable resource for helping kids with LD/ADHD develop confidence.

When I began mentoring for ETE, I jumped in and hoped for the best. I didn't really have any experience as a mentor; I just knew what it felt like to be a kid who struggled, both academically and socially, and I hoped that would be enough to enable me to connect with and help my first mentee.

Dario was a fifth grader who had been held back a year. Even if he hadn't been retained, he would have been a big kid for his grade. He was from Cape Verde, about my size at a little over six feet, with broad shoulders. If you'd seen him playing basketball at the park, you might have thought he had everything going for him. He was good-looking and easily the best athlete on the court. However, when he was in class, he drew only negative attention because his thumb was in his mouth and he could barely be heard when he spoke.

"So how's school?" I asked as we sat awkwardly at the grammar school desks together. "Are you doing well?"

"Oh yeah," he told me. "Everything is great."

"How's your spelling? That was always rough for me."

"No problem," he said.

I quickly learned that working with Dario in a classroom wasn't going to be very productive—at least not initially. It was clear he felt weighed down in school, even when he was sitting at his desk without any teachers around. He was intensely aware of all the expectations he was unable to meet so he would just shut down. He didn't start owning up to his struggles until I revealed to him that I used to concoct the same kind of lies so people wouldn't know I had trouble spelling and reading.

I knew I needed to get Dario away from the classroom, so

we headed to the basketball courts. People thought he was a college freshman, which he loved. In school, he was seen only as a low-achieving fifth grader—a very hard identity to face every day. Being mistaken for a college student planted a seed in his mind that college was a possibility for him.

By going to the basketball courts, Dario got away from his demons for a little while. As we shot free throws, we fought some of the negative messages he had been absorbing for years. In addition to our time on the courts, we also completed a number of art projects together to spark more intimate conversations and create a feeling of safety and success that would translate to the classroom.

One project we put together was a superhero cape that demonstrated his strengths and weaknesses. Dario brainstormed "superhero strengths" to display on the outside of his cape, such as great basketball player, amazing friend to the underdogs in school, and creative writer. The things he struggled with, such as reading, focusing in class, and talking to teachers were on the inside. The cape mapped out his identity as a learner.

I asked him a lot of questions—When does your mind work well? When does it work poorly?—and we figured out what success felt like to him and what *he* believed enabled him to be successful. I also helped him see it wasn't his fault he had not become the best speller or wasn't able to sit still for hours at a time.

When Dario was able to look at his challenges in light of

his "superhero strengths," he began to open himself up to learning again and bring some of the self-esteem he had on the basketball court into the classroom. He began to see that his strengths were indeed formidable, and instead of just hoping his difficulties would go away, he could learn to do well with what he had. If one approach to learning wasn't working for him, he could try a different approach, and I would guide him through the process.

I benefited from our relationship as much as Dario did. I confronted some of my old fears from elementary school and stopped faulting teachers so much when their students floundered.

When I met first him, Dario desperately needed a mentor to gain self-confidence and resilience. He lived in a tiny house on Hope Street with his alcoholic mother and he slept on the couch. He'd never known his father. He *really* needed to be empowered.

When everyone in a family is struggling, it can seem as if there's not much that can be done for a kid like Dario. As his mentor, I constantly urged his family to let him create social capital in his life so he could be proud of something. He couldn't afford to have tutors come to his house, or to visit private learning specialists, but as he began to recognize his strengths, he gained confidence in the things he was actually good at and no longer allowed his challenges—both internal and external—to impede him.

Dario's family also began empowering him by giving him

chores that he wanted to do around the house. For example, when he discovered a love for cooking, his family allowed him to do the shopping and cook dinners instead of other things they might have asked him to handle. This made a huge impact: Dario ended up working in a restaurant at thirteen, and after high school, he attended Johnson & Wales, one of the best culinary schools in America.

Dario and I have stayed in touch over the years. Recently I asked him what our relationship provided that was most valuable. When Eye to Eye first began, we tried to teach reading. I thought Dario would say that instruction had been most helpful, but he didn't even mention it. Now I realize he would have learned to read without my help. What I did give him, he said, was praise and the belief that his efforts mattered. I also offered him a different vision for what school could be like, namely a place where he could grow and find a future filled with pride.

During my time as a mentor, I began to see a pattern: students with LD/ADHD either learned helplessness in the face of a one-size-fits-all education (and eventually dropped out of school), or they learned how to remove the stumbling blocks in their environment so they could use their innate intelligence to succeed.

As Dario's mentor, my first step was to take him out of his school environment, where he felt like an absolute failure, and challenge him on the basketball court, where he was a natural superstar. After fighting some of the negative messages he'd been hearing about himself in the classroom, we moved on to his house, the library, and other places to continue our conversation about how he could use his remarkable gifts to overcome hurdles in school.

While I've worked with many students like Dario who have developed their own ways to navigate the tough times they face as different thinkers, it's rare that kids don't feel some degree of shame about their LD/ADHD. Even with an early diagnosis and support, feeling different is tough on kids and can do a number on how they feel about themselves. Not surprisingly, when young people are overwhelmed by failure and shame, their ability to communicate suffers profoundly. Often they just shut down.

Clayton Christensen, author and business professor at Harvard, has written about the "job" that students are trying to do, and it's about much more than school or homework; it's feeling successful and having fun with their friends.

Given that, it's no wonder students with LD/ADHD struggle more than most—not only is it hard for them to feel successful in school, but they often stumble socially as well. Their frustration can lead them to take more risks than their non-LD/ADHD peers—with alcohol, drugs, and other kinds of dangerous behavior.

I see many kids who spin out of control at the point I had reached before I transferred to Schenck. They get typecast as bad kids and end up in a very different place than I did. In 2012, the UCLA Civil Rights Project reported that 13 percent of students with disabilities in kindergarten through twelfth grade were suspended during the 2009–10 school year, compared with 7 percent of students without disabilities.

The truth is, the majority of students with LD/ADHD never reach their full potential because by the time they're eighteen, they've received so much negative feedback on their school performance and often struggled so hard socially, they truly believe they're not good enough. This can keep them from getting the help they need, and sometimes make them act out in less-than-ideal ways.

To sum it up in one phrase: they are socially bankrupt.

The kids I work with face challenges their non-LD/ADHD peers conquer with ease. "The anxiety, fear, and confidence issues are much greater than the actual disability," says Vanessa Kirsch, the dyslexic mother of a dyslexic child. Even if kids are receiving the educational accommodations they need, it's hard for schools to cultivate the emotional intelligence that is essential to survival in the socially challenging world of children and teenagers. The emotional challenges of LD/ADHD are often the most damaging part—and the most hidden.

Overcoming Cured

For years I wanted to say I had "overcome" my dyslexia and ADHD. No one ever told me what this meant, exactly, but I knew I wanted it. After all, I had learned that dyslexia and

ADHD were biologically based and that my brain would not change. I learned that "remediation" was not meant to fix me, but to teach me differently. How to make sense of the conflicting messages was beyond me.

Nevertheless, when I went off to college I thought that perhaps, wrapped within my acceptance letter from Brown, was the false promise that I had somehow finally overcome my dyslexia and ADHD. Statistics said I would not graduate from the tenth grade. In fact, throughout my education, many people said to me implicitly and explicitly that I would never be college material. So unless Brown had made a mistake (and deep down I was always slightly worried they might have) I charged off to the Ivy League and imagined I was *cured*!

A number of curses are wrapped up in this concept of *cured*. I had spent eighteen years learning to work with my dyslexia and ADHD. In some ways, my dyslexia and ADHD had become my close friends, part of how I introduced myself and got to know my teachers. My college acceptance was not in spite of my dyslexia and ADHD but *because* of it: even my application was about my dyslexia and ADHD.

However, when I went to Brown in the fall of 1998, it was before Apple's "Think Different" campaign and the Coordinated Campaign for Learning Disabilities' "Not All Great Minds Think Alike" public service announcement. At best, I would speak of dyslexia and ADHD in the abstract, something I got over—like chicken pox. My different thinking was not yet fully part of my identity.

One thing I was certain of, however, was that I belonged in Education Studies. Because I had struggled throughout school and recently *overcame* my LD/ADHD, I felt I could learn to be a great teacher. Plus, my number one role model was my mother, a teacher for decades who had instilled in me the value of education. So one of the first classes I chose delved into education theory, practice, and pedagogy.

Professor L was a highly sought-after professor in the education department with a reputation for pushing her students. Nervous as hell, but bold as only naive freshmen can be, I walked into her office during my first week in college to talk my way into one of her advanced classes.

As someone with LD/ADHD, I felt as though I had been studying education my whole life. Like an athlete watching replays of the big game to learn how to improve, I had pored over every moment of my schooling. I was the puzzle piece that did not fit into the puzzle; that's why I wanted to work so hard in education. My dyslexia and ADHD gave me that. But as I tried to talk my way into the advanced class, I didn't mention these points. Perhaps that's what it meant to be cured, I thought.

When she questioned why I should be able to skip the intro classes, I cited material of hers, hoping to get on her good side. She paused, intrigued. I then challenged some of her thinking, showing that I was ready to deal with hard ideas. Finally, realizing I was not leaving without a yes, she agreed to let me into her advanced seminar—as long as I could keep up.

I was very excited for our first writing assignment and quickly realized that my usual challenges were less daunting when studying what I loved. I also was being smarter about my schoolwork. I had already looked ahead at the syllabus and skimmed all the books, since I knew it would be tough for me to read each week's assignment thoroughly. I did read the book for my big paper from cover to cover, though, so I was eager to write and started well before the deadline for the assignment, another new approach for me.

Deep in the basement of the library, distraction free, I wrote what I thought was a very solid paper. I still used certain accommodations, like my laptop's spell-check, but so did everyone else by this time. I even asked my new roommate to read my paper over, but he only made content corrections. I felt like a new student. Even better, I had tackled the topic of dyslexia without telling one person about *my* dyslexia.

After I turned in the paper, I couldn't stop thinking about my grade. I became certain it was my best work ever and that it would legitimize me in the professor's eyes. Several weeks passed, then Professor L handed me my masterpiece. At the top of the page in red ballpoint pen was *A / See Me*.

As I awaited the accolades I had been striving for my whole life, Professor L began.

"David, you wrote a wonderful paper, full of interesting arguments that were well cited. But . . ."

The word *but* hung in the air for what seemed like an eternity. She reached into her desk and pulled out a copy of my paper. I noticed for the first time that it was covered in red ink. I was on the brink of tears, not because of my spelling and grammar mistakes but because of the word *but,* which in my mind completely negated the positive.

"Your spelling and grammar are nowhere near college level," she explained. When she asked why I had consistently spelled *to* "t-o" even if I was referring to the number or *also,* I tried my usual joke.

"I figured I had a 33 percent change of getting it right."

But the charade was up. The look on her face said she did not find my joke particularly funny. So I confessed.

"I'm dyslexic, and I can't tell the difference between all those *tos.*

She looked at me kindly and said, "No problem. Just take this paper to the writing center and have it proofread. Fix it up and you'll be all set."

No problem? *This is a* big problem, I thought. What happened to overcoming my dyslexia?

I left, fuming. My roommate *had* proofread my paper to avoid this very dilemma. I stormed back to my dorm and when my roommate came home, I plopped the paper, bleeding with red marks, in front of him.

"You were supposed to help me where spell-check left off! I'm dyslexic!"

He struggled not to giggle. Then a chuckle slipped out. Then, full-on tears ran down his face with explosive laughter to match.

"I'm dyslexic too!"

It didn't take long before my anger melted into laughter as well. Since we still don't have a secret handshake for dyslexics, we had both missed the obvious.

Before I submitted my paper, I should have either told my roommate about my dyslexia or found someone whose role was clear—someone in the writing center, for example. It wasn't the first or last time I made this mistake, however. In a bad habit I've come to call *dating for spellers,* during my first few years at college, I tried to date English majors or other women I suspected might have strong editing skills. I don't recommend this approach—it didn't make for very good dates *or* very well edited papers.

At the writing center, I found someone without dyslexia to proof my paper. I abandoned the idea that my dyslexia prevented me from being able to do my best and from asking for the help I needed. I wrote my next paper on stigma and the impact of language such as *but* and *and*. It was titled "Dyslexic ~~but~~ *and* Smart."

Words matter. While Professor L was incredibly supportive and understanding, in my mind, her very instinctual use of the word *but* undercut my achievement. I couldn't even absorb the praise she gave me on that paper because all I could see were the red marks and my failure to dot my i's and cross my too's. In the gentlest of ways, I shared these feelings with her over coffee one day after class.

Though kids get blamed for speaking before they think,

parents and teachers are often guilty of the same behavior. It's human nature. I know we can sometimes go too far in the other direction as well—being *overly* conscious of our language, to the point where we become paralyzed. But there's a happy medium, a place where the praise can get through and not be diminished by criticism. That criticism is equally important. I needed to learn how to proofread my papers more effectively. If my professor had let my grammatical mistakes slide, then my work would have continued to be marred by errors.

If we make an effort to always start with the positive, to put the good first, then students will be in a better place to receive criticism. Professor L had done exactly that; even so, I was devastated by my failure, rather than buoyed by my success. And I had a fairly healthy ego. Imagine a more fragile student, one who hasn't experienced many A's or science awards or home runs of any kind. Every bit of progress is a milestone.

For all of us, shortcomings are plentiful. Victories? Not so much. So celebrate even the smallest victory whenever you get the chance. And turn down the volume on the disappointments. Everyone will be grateful.

Right Ally, Right Time

Choosing allies is an art. So is being one. If you're a parent, you are your child's number one ally—but not for every situation. Knowing when to be which kind is an essential skill when trying to support different thinkers. Sometimes, you need to be outspoken, noisy, noticeable. Other times, it's best to remain behind the scenes, anticipating and preparing, like the sweepers who smooth the ice for their teammate in curling.

My father was a tremendous ally when I needed someone to decipher my biology text. But if he had tried to edit my papers . . . we both would have seen red, and I would have lost faith in him as an important ally. Be a parent first. And realize that you aren't always the right ally—in fact, you can damage your relationship with your child by trying to help when you should step aside.

Stepping aside doesn't mean abandoning your child; it means honestly considering whether or not you are the right person to provide what is needed. Sometimes you can be an ally by locating the top resources, or by recognizing that the help your child is receiving isn't working.

So let's talk about some of the ways you can be a good parent/ally to your different thinker. Again, it starts with the basics. In addition to language, environments have an enormous impact on different thinkers, as we've discussed. Take a look around your home. Is it messy, noisy, chaotic? Or does everything have its place—or at least an *assigned* place, a goal to shoot for when trying to keep track of school appointments and textbooks and soccer uniforms and phone chargers. Surroundings matter, especially to kids with attention issues. While you can't always ensure that they will be enveloped by a river of calm, do what you can to limit the noise, the mess, the uncertainty, the . . . instability. Their brains will thank you.

Many of these ideas seem so simple as to be obvious or easy. They're not. Being a great ally requires great thought— really understanding your different thinker and exactly what will enable him to access his strength and talents.

I have a friend who is a new mother. She's also one of the most disorganized people I know. Yet somehow, with her child, she is as structured as a Marine Corps colonel.

"I have to be," she told me. "Even if my office is in chaos, I make sure that Sophia's room is a peaceful oasis. And that naptime and bedtime are the same every day. Just don't ask me when my car's oil needs to be changed."

We all have our strengths and weaknesses—even you folks who aren't different thinkers. Knowing them is essential, especially if you want to provide the best support possible. So if your housekeeping skills are less than stellar, think about asking for help. Similarly, if you're not a great speller, do not offer to proof your child's homework assignment. Protect your relationship—and the trust that comes with it—at all costs. And learn to delegate when necessary.

Self-awareness is key in all you do, but particularly as you try to support your child with LD/ADHD. Understanding what kind of thinker as well as what kind of parent you are helps define your role and guides your decisions. There's a difference between helping and teaching: you won't always be able to do both—you may not be able to do either on occasion. That's when you may need to ask teachers, mentors, or tutors to step in.

Sometimes, it's more important to remind your child to do his homework than it is to help him do it. We've all heard about the value of teaching someone to fish versus handing them a bunch of canned tuna. Yet with our kids, such a hands-off approach can be hard to implement, especially if they're struggling.

In that struggle is the chance to learn and to grow, something that we all aspire to for our kids. During my senior year at Brown, I almost didn't finish my thesis, but my adviser insisted on it. If she hadn't—and if I had taken the easier path—I wouldn't have believed that I could. The confidence I gained in that effort was perhaps the biggest prize of my education. Don't rob your kids of the chance to acquire such a priceless gift: namely, trust in themselves.

There may be times when kids need to realize they have made mistakes and your job as ally shifts. Early in my high school career at Galloway, I was working on an eight-page world history paper, the longest assignment I'd ever had and a daunting task for any student, never mind a kid with dyslexia and ADHD. I wrote the entire paper on our home computer, which was a godsend in many ways except for one: it didn't save automatically like today's computers do.

You know what comes next. In my ADHD negligence,

rushing to complete the assignment the night before it was due, we had a power surge and the paper vanished, instantly, with no way to recover a single paragraph. I hadn't hit *save* even once.

I was old enough to understand the consequences but young enough to totally break down like only a kid can.

My mother was by my side during this debacle, as teacher and parent. She very easily could have tried to console me by relating this disaster to something similar that had happened to her, but we both would have known it wasn't the same. School was never hard for my mother; in fact, she had excelled academically. So if she had said, "I know how you feel . . ." I wouldn't have believed her.

Instead, she did the best thing possible: she ran me a bath. Then she lifted my sad little body up off the floor and led me to the tub, where I stayed for half an hour. And you know what? I regained my sanity.

The next day, I faced my teacher and told her what had happened. My mother hadn't stayed up all night to help me rewrite the paper and she also didn't send a note to my teacher. She let me bear the consequences of my actions. And that was a more important lesson than anything I may have learned in the paper. As I sat in the bathtub that night, I had no doubt I was loved. Sometimes, that's all a different thinker needs in order to move forward and face another day.

Allies can lead kids to many different lessons. Some are

painful, some are uplifting. All of them, however, should help kids grow into their best selves.

Hovering

In recent years, parents have come under fire for doing *too* much for their kids. *Helicopter parents* are universally scorned and often blamed for the shortcomings of their progeny. Parents insist that they're only doing what's best for their kids, but forget that there are lessons to be learned in the struggle; even kids with LD/ADHD benefit from fighting their own battles sometimes.

Your help has to be in response to your child's situation and balance her need for support with her need for competence. Hold back your urge to help unless it's clear your child can't move forward without it. Even then, make sure you support her effort rather than negate or eliminate the need for it.

With time and practice, if you listen to your child and your own instincts, you can discover the proper proportions between too little and too much support. Listening is a lost art, one that doesn't always exist between parents and children. But kids have a pretty good sense of what they need, if only we adults could hear them.

My father knew what I needed without my asking him. Heck, I don't think I would have necessarily articulated much more than I did—that the textbook was hard, that I was behind in my reading, that I was struggling. But he listened. In that simple act, he heard what I needed. And voilà, my science book on tape! When I lost my history paper, my mother knew intuitively what would help me most. That, too, is a kind of "listening" and one that requires some courage and faith.

I'm sure there are many more ways to "hear" and help your children, but some kids resist assistance—from you and anyone else who may try to lend a hand. They are their own little islands, determined to go it alone. Often, they even do pretty well on their own. Good for them.

But we all need help sometimes, and different thinkers are no exception. Sometimes islands need wheelchair ramps or the LD/ADHD equivalent. Fiercely proud children want to believe they can tough it out—an admirable trait in many ways. Then it becomes a parent's job to remind them of the value of just trying something new or different.

But change takes time, so make sure you build in a cushion of time for shifts to occur. Turning off the radio for an afternoon probably won't register positively. But keeping it off for a week or two may very well open your child up to the profound benefits of silence.

Sometimes you can sneak change in, perhaps by disconnecting the Internet before your child gets home from school or disabling the Xbox for a while. My mother had her own clever devices. During summers, after she picked me up from day camp, we'd sometimes go to a local magic shop where I learned how to perform new tricks. Other days we went to the library, where talented storytellers shared books with me.

These are just some quick examples of the subtle strategies we can all use to get our kids to do something different. Sometimes it even works the other way around, as our kids open us up to new ideas and ways of seeing ourselves.

Full Circle

Being an ally is not a one-way street. In the best cases, allies not only help others, they get something in return as well, whether it's a simple hug or a life lesson. The following story of two moms and their daughters shows how much we can all learn from—and help—each other, regardless of who is supposed to be helping whom.

Starting eighth grade was a big deal in Rosie's upstate New York public school. Homework increased, assignments were lengthier, and students were given more responsibilities. Rosie hoped someone could guide her through this big step in school, but she didn't know where to find her. Her mother, Jill, knew she had to let Rosie make this leap on her own, but still, she worried.

The school psychologist's office was next door to the principal's in Rosie's school, which was no more immune to the challenges of different thinkers than any other place, so there was frequently a revolving door between the two offices. Rosie, a well-behaved kid, was unsure why she had been summoned to the psychologist's office, where three years prior she had been diagnosed with LD/ADHD.

"Next week, we'd like you to join a new mentoring program called Eye to Eye," the psychologist informed her, "and you can meet cool college kids and work on art projects together. What do you think?"

"That sounds great," Rosie said, excited to work with older kids on her favorite hobby.

At nearby Hobart and William Smith Colleges, Shena Vagliano was ready to take on the world. In many ways, she already had; leaving New York City for boarding school as a sixteen-year-old, she was not afraid to make choices that would challenge her. She planned to finish college in three years instead of four so she could start to make a difference in the world, seeing no reason to pause in her ambition.

While everything had been highly structured in boarding school, when that structure vanished at college, Shena began to have a hard time focusing, so she met with the disability service staff and was diagnosed with ADHD. She spent the next month dissecting all her accomplishments and failures, trying to understand what kind of impact this "disorder" might have had on her life.

She decided to tell only her roommate about her diagnosis—if only to explain why she was taking "crazy pills." She quickly broke that rule and shared her secret with her best friend, Alice, the ETE coordinator. Before she knew it, Shena had agreed to join the program and mentor a girl with ADHD named Rosie.

At the first meeting for mentors, a pile of fidgets—a squish ball, a Rubik's cube, some Play-Doh—were in the center of the table. Nobody said a word and nobody touched the fidgets. Shena looked at the squish ball. Throughout her senior year, she had squished one just like it. The first task was to complete a survey, which began with the question *How do you spell success?*

"I was told there would be no spelling here," one student cracked. Two hours later, Shena had broken her rule about not sharing her ADHD identification fifteen more times as she began to understand she was a part of a hidden minority that was about to change the life of Rosie and her peers.

When Shena and the other mentors showed up at Rosie's school, Rosie was wearing her favorite hot pink jumpsuit. Shena had been told a bit about her mentee but not that she loved hot pink or that her dream was to be a cosmetologist. The two girls spent the session making a plaster cast of a handshake, representing their pact to work together. As they began to get to know each other, Shena searched for words to describe her ADHD experience. Rosie seemed to understand the meaning of ADHD better than Shena did.

Weeks passed and project after project gave Rosie and

Shena much to discuss. Together, they invented a magic tool that would help Rosie do better in school; at the touch of a button, it would organize all her assignments and magnetically collect her pencils. In the group mural project, each student wrote a truth about him- or herself in graffiti on a paper wall. Rosie wrote "I have trouble staying focused." Shena wrote "me too," and then they both sketched pictures of their favorite fidgets.

As the end of the school year approached, Shena asked Rosie how she could help her feel successful.

"I want to get on honor roll, high honor roll really. If I make honors, my mom's going to let me dye my hair hot pink. If I get high honors, then she's going to dye her hair too!" Shena thought about everything her mother had done for her, including letting her go to boarding school. But she had stopped short of dying her hair pink.

"How can I help?" Shena asked.

"You already have!" Rosie replied. And Rosie had certainly helped Shena become more comfortable with her own LD/ADHD. She wondered how a five-foot-tall eighth grader had enabled her to forget her shame and if the gift she had given Rosie could ever be as significant.

Shena stayed on campus that summer to take some extra classes. She was still set on graduating early and now that she better understood how she learned best, she was on track. One day as she pulled into the local grocery store, she noticed two tiny people with pink hair. Later, as she loaded her cart, Shena kept seeing hot pink out of the corner of her eye, but each time she turned to look, the double flash of pink vanished.

Finally, as she waited in checkout, there was Rosie, resplendent in her hot pink hairdo. Next to her was a woman in her midforties, also sporting a hot pink hairdo. High honors indeed!

I first heard this story almost four years after it happened. Rosie's mother, Jill, chose to celebrate whatever Rosie wanted and did whatever she could to make her dreams possible. "I never cared if Rosie was the best in class," Jill told me, "as long as she pushed herself to be *her* best. My job was to help her. Even if that meant dying my hair hot pink."

Jill's words were almost exactly the same as those of Shena's mother, Barbara. "When Shena was four," Barbara shared, "her pediatrician told me to help her however she wanted and then stay out of the way. I have been doing that ever since and she is changing the world."

When she was younger, Barbara was known for her "high jinks." After learning about Shena's diagnosis, she was inspired to get tested herself. When she was told that she too had ADHD, she stood proudly alongside her daughter.

"My mom is definitely my hero," Shena told me. "She will never just accept where she is in life—she always tries to think about why she does things. 'Think through your actions,' she tells me, which is an interesting thing for someone with ADHD to say, given that it's known to make people impulsive."

Shena went on, "She was better able to reflect on her marital issues after her diagnosis, and now she and my father are back together almost twenty years after their divorce." In addition to becoming closer to both her daughter *and* her ex-husband, Barbara has discovered a larger community; she was one of eight LD/ADHD artists-in-residence at ETE who helped design the 2012 ETE curriculum, one of our most successful to date.

The similarities between Jill and Barbara are not unusual. They support their kids to the end of the earth. What is unusual is the impact Shena and Rosie had on each other and even more so, how they affected their mothers. Rosie told her mother exactly what she needed in terms of support, a crazy act of faith. With a five-dollar bottle of hair dye, Jill solidified her place as an extraordinary mother. By redrawing her own story, Shena changed her mother and together they discovered a brand-new world.

So don't be surprised if by becoming an ally, you wind up with hot pink hair and a whole new perspective on life. Not only will you earn the gratitude of a different thinker, but you may just learn something about yourself as well.

Chapter 8

BECOME AN ADVOCATE

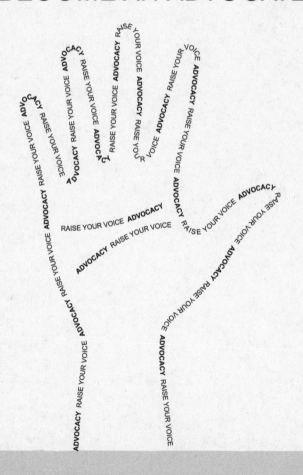

We need to encourage these kids to believe in themselves because if they are taught to, they will.

—Carol Moseley Braun, former U.S. senator and ambassador, dyslexic

There's no question that we all need allies, but sometimes we need advocates as well. An advocate is anyone who takes action or speaks up for someone whose needs aren't being met. For different thinkers, this can be a parent, teacher, mentor, or friend. At some point, it should also be the different thinker herself.

I've talked a lot about how to uncover tools that help those with LD/ADHD thrive in the classroom and beyond. This chapter discusses the best ways to acquire those tools. That's where advocates step in. Not only do advocates often know exactly what we need, but they also know how to get it.

Avatar Advocates

Let's start with some advocacy basics. Our protagonist is Jack, a seventh-grade boy in public school who has been diagnosed with dyslexia and ADHD. He's currently in a mainstream middle school where he gets extra help from the school's resource center three days a week. His mother made sure Jack's teachers and the resource center staff read his IEP. She also advocated for the center to hire someone trained specifically to work with dyslexic students.

Jack's an original thinker, but organization and punctuality are not in his tool kit. So he and his advocates color coded all his school materials—blue for science, red for math, green for English—and made sure that his notebooks, book covers, and folders matched. That way, he can quickly grab what he needs in the morning without wasting time. He also has two sets of books—one for home and one for school. Finally, he has two lockers at school—one for books and papers, and the other for everything else—coats, hats, lunch.

Just for fun, we're going to follow Jack through a typical day, starting from the moment he wakes up. There are actually several moments when Jack wakes up, since he has a hard time with transitions. First, his phone alarm goes off. After he hits snooze and falls back asleep, a groovy white light on his globe clock radio gets brighter and brighter, accompanied by the adrenaline-pumping tunes of his favorite band, which always put him in a good mood.

He had to advocate for the globe—his parents both thought it was unnecessary, given that he already had a cell phone and a perfectly good digital clock radio. But Jack convinced them that hearing his favorite band and being hit by the happy white light of the globe really made his entry into the day easier. His parents finally relented after he committed to walking their golden retriever every day when he got home from school.

He lingers in bed for a while—maybe a bit too long, and by the time the globe gets to the second song on the play-list, Jack's mom knocks on his door to let him know he has twenty-five minutes until he has to catch the bus. Every time he misses the bus, he loses five dollars from his weekly allowance of twenty bucks. Today is a Wednesday, and so far, Jack's allowance is intact.

Determined to keep it that way, Jack throws his feet over the edge of the bed and tries to get moving. He's already packed his book bag the night before to save time, as well as figured out what he's going to wear—never too difficult since he's a polo shirt and khakis kind of guy. Jack's mom helped him come up with these two time-saving strategies after seeing him struggle to get organized at seven A.M. day after day. She also makes sure he has plenty of clean polo shirts so there's never a fashion crisis.

After a shower and a quick but healthy breakfast of oatmeal (a slow-burning carbohydrate that's low in sugar—Jack's mom keeps an eye on his sugar intake since too much makes him crash), Jack is out the door, on his way to meet the bus. Last year, the bus route was painful: Jack's house was the second stop in the morning, a full hour earlier than it is this year.

Again, Jack has his mother to thank. She approached the bus line and suggested that they end at Jack's house. Next year, they'll return to the early schedule, but by then his sister can drive him to school. His mother's effective advocacy bought him a few more zzz's and bought her household a bit more early-morning peace.

By now, I think you're starting to get the picture as to how advocacy works, even in the simplest of ways. If you see something that might help your child without inconveniencing others, try it out, whether it's an inspiring piece of new technology or a later wake-up call. It's also a good idea to include your child in the process. In Jack's case, he stood to benefit from some changes and suggestions and was also willing to make a sacrifice to achieve his desires. In this way, he learned about both advocacy and personal responsibility.

When you advocate for your kids, don't leave them out of their own life choices. The more kids are invested, the more likely they'll adhere to commitments and honor promises. Otherwise, they might expect that you'll always be there to bail them out or fight for their best interests. As we all know, the world does not work that way.

Good advocacy is a balancing act; you must recognize what your child is able to do for himself and what he needs help achieving. Regardless, it's important to maintain an open dialogue throughout so that your child understands why you're seeking certain accommodations or the reasoning behind other choices and decisions. Before I started at Galloway, my mother met with my teachers to explain that I'd be using a computer and how it helped me learn better. She still made it *my* responsibility to speak to each of my instructors, however, which kept me invested in my learning plan.

Begin your journey at home, where you can see the impact certain decisions have, and together, you and your child can map out a way of working that suits both of you. Maybe your child's educational evaluation has revealed that he'd benefit from extra time or additional breaks on tests. This is something you both can advocate for. Perhaps your daughter has been assigned a window seat in her English class, but she knows that the distracting view is limiting her ability to pay attention. She can advocate for herself by explaining her situation to her teacher and asking for a new seat.

Too often, parents forget that a child is at the center of their battles, which become more about them than their kid with LD/ADHD who needs help. Don't let that be you: become a team. To quote an African proverb: *If you want to go fast, go alone. If you want to go far, go together.*

How far different thinkers can go depends to a large extent on the abilities and enthusiasm of the advocates and allies in their lives. While advocacy may start at home, it can extend far, far beyond to the local, state, and even national levels. But first, different thinkers have to learn to advocate for themselves.

Finding Your Voice

The most important kind of advocacy will always be the kind your child does for herself. Then she becomes the essential core of an unstoppable team, a team guided by her own needs and abilities, empowered by every triumph and learning from every failure without losing hope.

The first step in being able to advocate for yourself is to find your voice and learn how to ask for what you need. In essence, to speak up for what you're not getting.

This isn't always easy, especially for kids—and in particular for kids with LD/ADHD, who can be so discouraged and ashamed that they can't even look people in the eye when they talk. When I was growing up, my best friend, Michael, literally had to learn how to speak loudly enough to be heard, a fitting metaphor for the struggles of many kids with LD/ADHD.

Before Michael and I met, my teacher suggested that we spend some time together, telling our mothers we were born to be friends. Michael was by all measure the strong silent type. While I often held court at recess, telling jokes and doing tricks, Michael stood to the side quietly. He had wavy blond hair that he groomed to lie in front of his eyes to avoid eye contact. I reached out to Michael a couple of times, but he seemed content to walk his own path and commanded a silent respect from all of us as a result.

A date was arranged when Michael would come over to my house, but neither of us was overly excited. We had both matured a bit from the independence Schenck instilled in its students and suspected something contrived was afoot.

We were quickly surprised, however, by how much we shared. He was the first person to understand my struggles, and I appreciated his as well. We talked for three days straight.

Although we had faced similar emotional barriers, to the outside world we were very different people. My peers often told me to hush up when I talked too much, while Michael was encouraged to speak up. I preferred learning by dissecting topics through lively conversation. Michael was a hands-on kind of guy. I think sand taught him to spell; he told me he had traced the outlines of hard words in the sand over and over again.

By the end of seventh grade, we had become new students—confident readers and spellers, capable of using strategies to address our ADHD that allowed us to participate in class and do our homework. We had hit the lottery with our social capital reserves and were ready to take on the challenges mainstream education might throw at us. For this reason, in what may not be the best business model but is certainly good practice for their students, the Schenck staff advised that we move on to new schools.

It was clear that the world out there was very different from our little school. It wasn't built for us, but if we asked (nicely but firmly), we could get what we needed to succeed. The last task that remained was to become better self-advocates. With my loquacity and energetic spirit, I was built to advocate for myself, but Michael was a different story. His shyness was a liability and he knew it. He was at a crossroads.

One afternoon when I arrived at his house, his mother directed me downstairs, where Michael was building something with a noisy drill. I had to scream to let him know I was there. He yelled back *hello* and I almost fell over. I had never heard him make a noise louder than a mouse squeak.

He took off the bright orange earmuffs he was wearing to protect his ears.

"Oh, sorry," he said in the quiet voice I had come to know and love.

"Wait, that was awesome!" I said. "Could you always do that?"

"I'm working on it."

He then confessed that he had spent the better half of his morning screaming in a field. His reticence was not something he was ashamed of nor did he know why he had always been so quiet. While he had fought many demons at Schenck and walked out the victor on almost every count, he knew he needed to literally find his voice if he wanted to be his best. The drilling was part of this; he was working on speaking above the sound. I offered my full support and even let him know I'd happily go scream in a field with him whenever he so desired.

Michael and I never again attended the same school, though we saw each other regularly after school and on weekends. When he went off to college in the Midwest and I in the

Northeast, we amassed huge phone bills staying in touch. We were in each other's weddings; our wives are now friends, our families, incredibly tight.

Michael had his first child a year ago. Weeks before Ethan was born, Michael asked me what we'd do if his son had a learning disability, a real genetic possibility. I told Michael we'd just take Ethan to a field and go from there.

Michael had known he was smart, but in order to guide his own education and the perceptions of those around them, he needed to give voice to that intelligence. That's the first step for all different thinkers. While parents may want to provide whatever we can as advocates and allies, the journey begins in the hearts and minds of the kids who are living the LD/ADHD experience.

Owning their difference and being able to speak up to get what they need is an essential part of the journey for all students with LD/ADHD, whether it's by asking for a new seat assignment or by standing in a field and screaming your guts out. That journey often begins by knowing yourself and how to ask for help.

Self-Advocacy

To most effectively self-advocate, different thinkers have to accept their limitations, otherwise they'll keep getting stuck. For me, that moment came when I finally headed to the writing center at Brown, after my professor pointed out that my atrocious spelling mistakes had made an otherwise excellent paper barely college material.

Not that I didn't still make the occasional mistake or slip back into thinking I was *done* with my LD/ADHD.

I spent my junior year abroad in Australia, where all my grades were pass/fail. *How hard can it be just to pass?* I thought. Because of this misguided confidence, I didn't bother to register with disability services. Big mistake. My final grade in psychology would be based on the midterm and final. I received a C on the midterm; good enough in my book to prevent me from worrying. For the final, I studied like "normal" kids, cramming three days before the test.

I failed.

Failing wiped out any credit for the course and would delay my graduation from Brown. With only one day before I was scheduled to leave, there was little time to explain my huge lapse in judgment to the professor, but somehow . . . I tracked him down in time and pleaded my case. Although he admonished me for not getting the proper accommodations in advance, he let me write a paper before I left that demonstrated my knowledge of the materials. Within forty-eight hours, I was on a plane.

My paper received a B+, a passing grade. Crisis averted!

Even though I knew my LD/ADHD would be a factor because of the way I would be tested, I had mistakenly assumed I could get C's and be okay. But when you have LD/ADHD, it's either an A or an F—that's how big the ocean is between having accommodations and not. In college, I needed good grades for my future, so I made sure to get the help I needed.

When I entered grad school at Columbia, I was tested in ways that worked for me—with papers and projects as opposed to in-class, timed exams. My time at Columbia was also for my own personal development; when I learned for the sake of learning, I was much more motivated, which made it easier and more enjoyable to get good grades. It was the first time in my life I received all A's—and the first time it didn't really matter.

You have to be vigilant when you have LD/ADHD; if you assume you're "fixed" or that the same rules apply to you as those that apply to everyone else, you may be surprised when you struggle and even fail. This is why it is so important to help students develop self-advocacy skills at an early age. Kids need to know how to speak up and ask for help—and that skill is one they'll use throughout their life, in college and beyond. To be an effective self-advocate, you must accept who you are.

Think about it: How can you stand up for yourself if you haven't accepted who you are? All we need to do is look at some of the great leaders in the history of civil rights and we can see that above all else, they were proud of who they were. In fact, many groups still fighting for equality use the word *pride* as an integral part of their efforts.

Own Your Differences

My mentee Ben was a shining example of a student who'd had every advantage a person with dyslexia and ADHD could have. He attended a private high school in New York City, his father was a psychologist, and his mother, a teacher. In many ways, Ben was the complete opposite of Dario from Cape Verde, my first mentee. When I met Ben and asked about his grades, he didn't feel the need to lie to me the way Dario had, because Ben actually had good grades. He seemed socially confident and incredibly knowledgeable on a variety of subjects. He also felt comfortable enough to announce to me that he had dyslexia and ADHD. I thought this was unusual. He said he'd been diagnosed at such a young age that he couldn't remember a time when he hadn't described himself as "a dyslexic and ADHD person."

The system was working for Ben. He had great accommodations and support in school as well as at home. Ben didn't need many of the skills I taught Dario. Yet Ben remained deeply ashamed of his identity as a person with LD/ADHD. He was surrounded by people who said he shouldn't feel ashamed and still he wondered how I could stand up in crowded auditoriums and claim dyslexia and ADHD as part of my identity.

Ben had created a virtual prison for himself, putting all kinds of restrictions on what he could and could not accomplish. He frequently used his LD/ADHD as an excuse for not even trying to do things he wanted to do. This happened partly because he was such a conscientious person; he was very aware of the rules, or "how things are done," and he wanted to please his parents and teachers so much that he'd become afraid of taking risks that might result in failure. As his mentor, I had to teach him to feel comfortable doing things in ways that weren't necessarily "how things are done."

We began by exploring some new accommodations. First, I gave Ben permission to use audio books. He hadn't allowed himself to read this way because he'd internalized the message that it was somehow a form of cheating. Next, I taught him how to skim his textbooks for important information; no one had ever taught him how to do this effectively even though it's a basic study skill all students should have. I also, eventually, pushed Ben out of his comfort zone by having him join me onstage at a few different high schools and colleges to speak about growing up with LD/ADHD. We prepared for our presentations together, and by the time it was his turn to speak in front of an audience, he was stretching into a direction where he absolutely could not fail.

Ben slowly began to see his learning disability—and himself—in a totally different light. He stopped thinking about LD/ADHD as negative traits that needed to be hidden and began to understand that, depending on his environment, his learning style could either help or impede him. If he wanted to succeed at things he'd been afraid to even try, he'd have to become proactive in creating new accommodations when existing ones failed him. He'd also have to give himself permission to break the rules sometimes and seek allies to support him.

While Ben had extraordinary support in place, he came up against many of the same roadblocks as my first mentee Dario did because he was traveling down the very lonely road of living by other people's rules and expectations, striving to fulfill other people's dreams. Mentoring taught him how to play by his own rules—to create new accommodations and know he wasn't cheating—and succeed.

He showed remarkable strength and aptitude when he was able to stand up in an auditorium full of college students and talk about his journey with an LD/ADHD. He proved to himself that he could own his learning process and be proud of how his mind works. As a result, he inspired his peers and felt as if he'd contributed something meaningful to his community.

In the end, even though Dario and Ben had radically different life experiences, they both became successful when they learned to be proud of who they are and how their minds work.

Acceptance is an ingredient in every different thinker's journey, from the moment when parents suspect there may be a problem as they notice their child struggling in school or reluctant to tackle homework or any other number of ways kids have of letting us know that all is not well. Then testing results require a certain amount of acceptance, as both parents and students adjust to their new understanding of learning issues. Accommodations often come with a period of adjustment as well. It takes time for students to accept alterations to their learning environment, whether it's a noticeable change like extra time on tests or assistive technology or a subtle aid like using color-coded binders.

But as I hope the stories in this chapter demonstrate, the more important kind of acceptance revolves around identity. Owning your different brain, with all its strengths and weaknesses, is paramount. If you don't accept—and even embrace—your brain, you're really limiting just how much you can achieve. What's more, there's less chance that others will be able to benefit from your triumphs if you don't allow them to be part of a greater LD/ADHD story.

Chapter 9

JOIN THE MOVEMENT

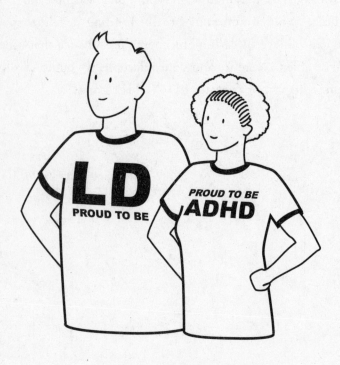

My dyslexia and my challenges
through school were the absolute
perfect training for an expedition.
—Ann Bancroft, polar explorer,
philanthropist, dyslexic

My first public speaking request as a "Proud Dyslexic" was at Schenck, my old middle school. Although I was touched the administration and teachers there thought I had accomplished something notable enough to inspire their students, the requirements for the gig were pretty low: I had graduated from high school. When your population drops out of high school twice as often as those without LD/ADHD, it's not tough to pass the bar for credentials that inspire.

As I got older and continued to "not drop out," I received more and more requests to speak. At first, I thought it was because I liked telling stories, but I soon realized that I was one of the few people willing to wear my LD/ADHD on my sleeve. This is not a metaphor, by the way. I often arrived at my speaking engagements wearing shirts that said THIS IS WHAT DYSLEXIA LOOKS LIKE.

By the time Eye to Eye had reached the national stage, I was receiving more speaking requests than I could manage. I was encouraged that my story and that of ETE seemed to hold such promise and potential for folks hoping to understand LD/ADHD, but two problems quickly arose.

First, I needed to pick my time away from the office carefully so as to best serve the movement ETE was helping to build. Second, mine is not the only story that matters. In fact, my story is only valuable if it inspires others to speak.

Stories That Matter

I encourage all the people I meet to tell their LD/ADHD stories. Whether it's the story of their journey, their LD/ADHD child's, or their LD/ADHD friend's—we must talk about our collective experiences to change misconceptions. I recognize that not everyone is ready to share their experience in a compelling and instructive way: it takes practice, confidence, training, time, and more practice, which happen to be core competencies of ETE. That's why I knew our student/mentors would be up for the challenge.

So in October 2011, ETE started the Think Different Diplomats, a group of two dozen students who became ambassadors of what's possible with dyslexia and ADHD. Their sole purpose is to dispel the idea that anyone could ever be so disabled that they couldn't learn. As one of my favorite ETE students puts it, "Imagine if someone didn't think you could learn . . . and you did anyhow."

The Think Different Diplomats worked on how best to tell their stories and be confident in front of a crowd during an "ADD tour" that crisscrossed the United States, dispelling myths and putting a face on an often invisible experience. In partnership with a wonderful peer organization, the National Center for Learning Disabilities (NCLD), ETE brought the Diplomats to Capitol Hill to help our politicians better understand the LD/ADHD experience.

We arrived just when the ESEA (Elementary and Secondary Education Act), also known as No Child Left Behind, was under reauthorization. We worried that lawmakers might make decisions that affected students with disabilities without talking to many students with disabilities. This would not be very surprising to us given that to many people, dyslexia and ADHD are invisible and that very little organizing of youth with LD/ADHD had occurred before ETE came along.

One revision being considered was no longer requiring individuals with disabilities to participate in high-stakes testing. Although I am not a fan of high-stakes testing and I'm sure there are some dyslexic and ADHD students who'd opt out if they could, we felt that not holding people with disabilities to the same high standards as everyone else would send the wrong message and be a step backward. Enter the Diplomats.

As a 501(C)(3) charity, ETE cannot lobby. We are also not in the business of lobbying; we are in the business of storytelling. So we came to the Hill with one mission: to put a face to LD/ADHD. Escorted and guided by our allies from NCLD, we met with a variety of lawmakers. This may have been the first time young LD/ADHDers had ever gone to the Hill in this way, to speak for themselves and to share their stories, their challenges, and their vision for the future.

Kevin from Hobart and William Smith Colleges, a sharp guy in a full suit, starched shirt, and Windsor knot in his tie, told Senator Michael Bennet of Colorado that his LD/ADHD helped him understand exactly how he learned, which was the key to his success.

Next was Isaiah of Columbia University, whose ADHD made him forget his tie but didn't impinge on his eloquence. Isaiah spoke of growing up in Harlem with a single mother, who had been his biggest advocate, but who was too afraid of the potential stigma to get him diagnosed. Isaiah talked about the kids in Harlem he was helping find the confidence to own their LD/ADHD so they could get the help they needed sooner.

Last up was Jeremy, a former football player who exudes kindness despite his imposing heft. Jeremy was as confident as anyone I had ever met, so I was shocked when I first learned that ADHD was the root of his academic struggles. If even I could misjudge so easily, no wonder others failed to recognize members of the LD/ADHD community. As a nineteen-year-old Wesleyan student, Jeremy was still learning to manage his

ADHD. He had forgotten his belt, so he untucked his shirt to cover it up. He had also forgotten his tie, but he had ironed his collar to near perfection.

What he had not forgotten was his poise and his story, something he took with him everywhere. A long silence filled the room as Jeremy made eye contact with everyone, finally locking eyes with Michael Bennet, who had been the superintendent of Denver Public Schools and now sat on the Education Committee. If anyone would be sympathetic to our cause, it was him.

"Senator, you have heard the stories of my peers, and I have had a lot of the same experiences," he began. "I came here today to let you know that I am proud of my brain with its gifts and its flaws. *That* is what it means to be a successful person with LD/ADHD."

As Senator Bennet felt the power of what had just been said, he raised his right hand and with equal power added, "I just want you to know that this U.S. senator is dyslexic and proud of his brain, with its gifts and its flaws."

My mouth dropped open in amazement and I spoke for the first time all day.

"I'd just like to say this is a moment worth noting," as I looked around the stately office, American and Colorado flags hanging on the wall. "Here we are, five people with LD/ADHD, all owning our brains. Celebrating our differences. Divided perhaps in age, but united in experience. All of this in a U.S. senator's office. Thank you, Senator."

As soon as my ADHD impulse left my system, I realized I had forgotten someone. There was a sixth person in the room: Jonathan, Senator Bennet's chief of staff. I immediately backtracked and tried to explain that I hadn't meant to leave him out, that he was an important ally, essential in setting up the day.

"You didn't leave me out," he interrupted. "I'm dyslexic too!"

"You are?" Michael said.

"Absolutely!"

Weeks later, the referendum to ESEA was abolished, making it clear we would not expect less of LD/ADHD students. While I recognized that we still faced many battles, at least we know that Jonathan and Michael are on our side.

Though this story features a U.S. senator, thousands of stories just like it play out across the country every day. As people become more and more open about their LD/ADHD, attitudes and perceptions will change. We will also continue to transform how we teach, how we learn, and what we expect of our students. For those reasons alone, being open about our LD/ADHD is an essential part of the journey all of us are making as we try to build learning environments that work for everyone.

Beyond that, openly owning your LD/ADHD provides a great opportunity to join a community of different thinkers, people just like you *and* completely unique in the way they think, learn, and act in the world. Together, the LD/ADHD nation can accomplish many things, both for us and others. We stand on the shoulders of those before us who struggled to overcome bias and discrimination. We can never forget their work. But now it's our turn.

Strike Out Stigma

Strike Out Stigma was the brainchild of Shena, whom you read about earlier in the book and who went on to work in our national office as our director of engagement and communications. For LD/ADHD awareness month one year, we wanted to bring the ETE message beyond our immediate members. Shena suggested we form a street team and head out our front door to the crowds in Times Square.

Armed with posters and bullhorns and wearing T-shirts that announced THIS IS WHAT DYSLEXIA LOOKS LIKE, we decided to see how many people with LD/ADHD we could entice in an hour to take a picture with us, next to posters that said "People with ADHD are ~~lazy~~ determined" *and* "LD = ~~less~~ equally intelligent."

Though as a group we were all extremely comfortable talking about our LD/ADHD and owning our labels, as Shena said, it's a whole different thing when you're screaming it through a megaphone. Within a short time, though, dozens of people stepped up to talk to us or get their picture taken.

It was a great day and we all returned to the office energized and ready to continue our work on the front lines of the LD/ADHD movement.

Shortly after we posted a video of the day on our Facebook page, a group of mentors who met in ETE decided to take the street team one step further. They planned to drive, after they graduated from college that year, from San Francisco to Providence, Rhode Island, striking out stigma in cities nationwide.

"The three of us behind the road trip are poster children for living with LD/ADHD. We can show people a diagnosis is not an academic death sentence," Erica told me from her dorm room in Washington. "Our stories are a great counter-image to all the misperceptions about learning disabilities out there. We want to put ourselves in the public eye."

This was a brave move, considering that the first time Erica and her friends tried to Strike Out Stigma in San Francisco, it didn't go so well.

The three young women positioned themselves in a major tourist area on the Saturday before Christmas, announcing on a bullhorn that "having dyslexia doesn't mean you're stupid and ADHD doesn't mean you're lazy." Unlike the crowds in Times Square, however, a few rowdy onlookers began to harass them, tossing off insults and mocking their efforts. But instead of making the girls think twice about their summer road trip, it only strengthened their resolve.

"Before we started, we'd all had some experience with

stigma. With LD/ADHD, someone is bound to make a joke or say something without thinking," Erica acknowledged. "They'll say things like 'You're dyslexic? And you got this job?' as if my LD/ADHD had something to do with my IQ or my ability to work hard. They have no clue about the actual struggle, the invisible struggle, when you're crying at home over homework or staying up late to finish a project. So much of what we go through is private."

Putting a public face on what can so often be a private disability is part of the impetus behind Strike Out Stigma and all of ETE's awareness-raising efforts. Sure, we can pass as "normal" and never get noticed. That's a personal decision. But for those of us who are ready to stand up and be counted, there are many, many reasons to do so.

Opening Minds

Let me start with a story I still can't believe. When I was a grad student at Columbia, my adviser in dis/Ability Studies, the head of the program, had a visual impairment. It wasn't long before I learned she believed physical disabilities were more valid than learning disabilities. Whenever we spoke about the matter, she used the argument of my success against me; she had bought into the idea that a person with LD/ADHD wasn't supposed to be like me and that because I was succeeding, it proved I didn't have a disability.

But many of my successes had occurred because I had been

able to use accommodations—the same kind of accommodations that enable people with physical disabilities to access what able-bodied people take for granted. As I've said before, books on tape or voice recognition software are like wheelchair ramps for dyslexics, allowing us to get from point A to point B without dragging our brains up the stairs.

Perhaps I should have cited some of the amazing athletes who, despite tremendous physical limitations, manage to achieve feats of athletic prowess able-bodied people can only dream of. Through their resolve, dedication, and training, they do more with their "different" bodies than some able-bodied people even try, but not without accommodations. Are people with LD/ADHD who achieve great things academically or in the business world any different?

I never challenged my adviser in this way, but my frustration with her—shock and deep disappointment actually—were part of what drove me to help elevate awareness of learning differences. I'm grateful that through her negative example I was inspired to contribute to a positive change in how people with learning differences are perceived.

Though I, too, was once guilty of not recognizing my own people.

Back when I was still a budding magician on the preteen entertainment circuit, I performed at a nearby day camp one summer. My audience consisted mostly of seven- to ten-year-olds, and when I asked for a volunteer, a young girl named Rachel raised her hand. All went smoothly; I didn't lose any rabbits or fail to produce the requisite number of strange items from ears. But when I spoke to the camp director after my show, she was in tears.

"David, I don't think you realized it, but your volunteer assistant was mostly deaf," the director explained. "Today was the first time all summer she turned on her hearing aid. And the first time she smiled and laughed."

I was shocked. And something in me shifted.

I managed to track Rachel down soon after that and even performed at her birthday party. As I was contemplating what to do for the service portion of my bar mitzvah, I decided to perform at Rachel's school. She attended a public school exclusively for students with special needs, from hearing impairment to muscular dystrophy to, yes, learning and attention issues just like mine. For whatever reason, however, I completely failed to see myself as one of them, even though I was enrolled at Schenck—a school specifically for students with learning disabilities.

Instead, I grew increasingly concerned that "those kids" weren't going to understand my jokes or the magic. While I knew Rachel was smart, my biases had convinced me that the rest of the students weren't. I think because I had yet to see myself as part of a broader community of people with disabilities, I failed to recognize that these were *my* people.

Even when I had to make some minor alterations to my act—such as speaking more slowly so students would be able to understand me and to allow time for the sign language person to communicate, I still didn't see the parallels to my own life. These were simply accommodations—the same sort of accommodations I required in school to learn my lessons.

The show went off without a hitch and soon I developed a whole new audience for my act. But the real magic of that day was when I realized that these kids, far from being worthy of my pity or somehow different from me, were in fact being disenfranchised just as I had been. I still didn't make the connection that we were part of the same community in many ways, but I did see that they were as "normal" as anyone else, myself included. And far from feeling like a chore, this so-called community service project made me consider my own values and put myself in the place of those I was trying to serve.

Empathy. Sometimes it can make all the difference. Again I'll say that is why ETE is so successful. Because our mentors have so many shared experiences with their mentees, trust is easier to establish and mentors are more likely to become models of hope and inspiration. That's why it's so essential for those with LD/ADHD to come out and join our community.

Finding Our People

Parents can't be all things to their children, much as they might try. My mother could soothe me when our computer lost my paper, but she couldn't *relate*. My father, with his

ADHD, might have been better able to relate, but since he'd never really identified as ADHD, he could only try to help.

Allies and advocates are great and necessary parts of every different thinker's life. But it's also essential to have a few people who really know what it's like to walk around in the world and experience it differently than the majority of the population does.

Because LD/ADHD is contextualized around learning, not necessarily around community, having LD/ADHD can feel very isolating at times. If you're one of the few kids in a mainstream classroom who gets pulled out for extra reading help, you probably feel singled out in a way that's not very comfortable. Or you may decide to lurk in the shadows and not share your LD/ADHD status.

This secrecy may seem preferable to the potential stigma you might face if you were open about your LD/ADHD, but you also pay a price for hiding how you learn. You'll be less likely to learn with and from your peers with LD/ADHD, who are great resources for discovering unique accommodations. You'll also be less likely to tap into the LD/ADHD community outside of the classroom, where you'd be able to share experiences beyond those related to academics.

"One of the reasons I love being involved in Eye to Eye," one of our mentors told me, "is because it's fun! Most LD/ADHD times are *not* fun—they're secretive or revolve around schoolwork. Very little has to be said for us folks with LD/ADHD to connect. 'I'm dyslexic' says it all."

"We were not in the cheetahs, we were in the turtles" is how another mentor explained the connection LD/ADHDers instantly feel with one another. "There's nothing worse than feeling like you're the only person who can't finish a book. When you're with other people with learning issues, that's the norm—and it feels good not to be the exception for a change."

"Everyone gets distracted at some point in their day, but people who use that to claim they're ADHD are really annoying—and wrong," Shena shared with me recently. "When everybody thinks they have ADHD, it undermines what real ADHDers struggle with every day. I'm *jealous* of people who get sucked into a book."

These kinds of frustrations can only truly be understood by fellow LD/ADHDers. Finding your people not only helps you find solutions, but it also helps you avoid pitfalls and build resilience. It enables you to make better decisions, both in and out of the classroom. Most of all, connecting with other different thinkers *normalizes* LD/ADHD, a goal we should all help achieve.

Join the Club

What are some of the other perks of this nation of different thinkers? Do you get free sprinkles at Dairy Queen? Sadly, no. But I promise you there are other benefits.

When I was growing up, my mother had many wonderful friends, and I still marvel at the intimacy that arose from what appeared to me as trivial connections—cookie recipes and Hanukah party planning. Through the lens of my dyslexia and ADHD, I now see that they found a bond around their Judaism: the cookies and party planning were simply by-products or cultural artifacts that facilitated that bond and strengthened it through their heritage. While I don't think we will ever have an LD/ADHD cultural cookie, the more we own our LD/ADHD identities, the more we will find and create our own stories and cultural artifacts.

People with LD/ADHD have common values and bonds just like any other minority. When we hide these identities, we lose the joy of connecting around these similarities. Step into an LD/ADHD home, and you'll notice a few things right away. For one, you probably won't see many books lining the shelves. Those that are there either have never been opened (check the binding), are only half read (look for a bookmark in the first forty pages), or are completed and stand like trophies on display.

Maybe you'll spot a bulletin board or to-do list on the fridge. Chances are, it will be filled with a wide variety of unrelated tasks. Ask someone with ADHD how many projects they are currently working on and the answer is usually half a dozen or more (several that have been in process for months). Most are half done and as soon as one is completed, a few others have already taken its place. People with ADHD never check everything off their lists.

If this sounds familiar and you're the parent of a child with

LD/ADHD, you may be one of the millions of adults living with an undiagnosed learning difference or attention issue. Don't fret; my hope is that by reading this book, some of my stories and suggestions may not only help you do the right thing for your child, but they may help you as well.

I recently got to know a woman who's been a very successful advertising professional for decades. As a creative director, Leslie's stock in trade is images; she studied painting in college and also had a brief career as a photographer. But throughout her success, she was often dogged by a feeling that she was inferior in some ways to her peers, as she would stumble over her words in meetings and say the exact opposite of what she meant all too frequently. She didn't feel *stupid*, exactly, but she did walk around worrying that she had misspoken on business calls or was hesitant to contribute her thoughts during meetings.

In her late forties, however, she began to learn more about dyslexia and how it might play out in the workplace. As she did, she slowly began to believe that all her malapropisms and verbal gaffes were not a result of a less than impressive intellect, but rather of a differently wired brain. This gave her some solace in her hypercompetitive, high-stress job. But she never openly acknowledged that she was dyslexic; she kept that possibility in her back pocket as an explanation she could turn to when she was feeling less than confident.

Interestingly enough, Leslie also happens to be gay. That part of her identity, too, took her years to accept and even longer to be fully open about with others, especially coworkers. As gays and lesbians gained increasing acceptance, however, she became better able to share her orientation, to the point that it is now rarely an issue for her at all.

It wasn't until recently, however, that she was able to be open about her dyslexia. In fact, the way she announced it one day at work surprised even her.

"My assistant was reading a phone number for me and I had to ask her to repeat it several times," she explained to me. "Finally, I just blurted out, 'Can you just dial it for me? I'm dyslexic, you know, and I have a really hard time with numbers.' Several other members of my staff were standing nearby and all of a sudden, they stopped what they were doing and stared at me like my hair was on fire. I just smiled and went back to work like it was no big deal. I don't think I realized what I had done until I got home that night and told my partner."

One of the many great things about this story is that even though Leslie had never spoken about her dyslexia at work before, once she did, it was in a very matter-of-fact manner that completely disarmed her colleagues. But perhaps the biggest difference it has made is in how she sees herself.

"It hasn't come up since that day," she told me, "but now I don't feel like such an idiot when I can't spell something. All those years when I worried what people thought about me . . . it's so sad and such a phenomenal waste of energy."

Owning your label can take many forms. But acceptance

is the key to the whole process. If you accept who you are, owning your LD/ADHD is as simple as owning your brown hair or your freckles. It simply *is*.

Make Some Ripples

The remarkable effects of this kind of self-acceptance are too numerous to count; as my friend and colleague Marcus Soutra has said, it's like the ripples in a pond. When you accept your LD/ADHD, everyone around you is affected by your ease and comfort. They, in turn, are able to spread that grace to people they come in contact with, who repeat the process in their circles until the whole pond is shimmering with the ripples stemming from one person who has simply said "I am . . ."

I believe this is how you start a movement. If we make some ripples, they are bound to spread until the entire pond is alive with their energy. That's how ETE makes such a profound impact on every mentee, mentor, school, community, and organization it has touched. Because when one child develops the strength and resiliency to own his or her brain and all its glorious differences, then everyone around that child is changed.

That kind of organic change is at the heart of ETE's mission, but to right educational injustice across the country and destigmatize LD/ADHD, empower labeled individuals, and achieve equal opportunity for different learners, we need your help, help that can create a world where all learners are recognized. Not all *different* learners. *All* learners.

For the LD/ADHD movement, however, there is more to be done. In my work for ETE, I hear a lot of talk about an LD/ADHD rights movement. At best, I think we have a *nudgement*. Why do I believe this? Because even our biggest gatherings are small compared to what constitutes a real movement. We are still focused on the individual, not the masses.

My final request in these final pages is that you empower your child, empower yourself, then push a little further and make changing the world part of your values, because an empowered child and an empowered parent is all that it takes to change the world. We *have* the numbers: we are 20 percent of the population. When we consider our ripples—friends, teachers, politicians, CEOs, postal workers, and dog walkers we talk to every day who would be our allies if we only told our story—we are everyone.

Now is the time to speak up for our kids and all learners. The nascent lessons I have laid out in this book are just blossoming now, but in years to come, with your support of our kids, they will become ubiquitous. Every child who is empowered makes the path for the children behind him easier to follow.

I have every degree of faith that LD/ADHD struggles will be things of the past in a generation or two. I look forward to the day when this book serves a greater purpose as a paperweight or a historical object than as an LD/ADHD owner's manual. I hope this chapter remains, though, because what I am sharing is a timeless lesson.

LD/ADHD Is Here to Stay

Different thinkers aren't going anywhere. Today, specialized software transforms written texts into an audio format on smartphones, tablets, and computers. As a result of constantly evolving technology, many of our current battles will become less important as ways to learn change. But I am certain there will always be some segment of the population who will struggle with what is considered the "normal" way to learn.

At ETE, 80 percent of our staff is LD/ADHD while the 20 percent that is not balance our weaknesses. We try to hire different thinkers because it is important to act affirmatively. We also see the untapped value of different thinkers, who have enabled ETE to become such a successful and dynamic organization. When you have lots of different thinkers rolling around, however, you have to be ready to provide a wide array of accommodations.

The same technology that "cures my dyslexia" on my iPhone creates huge barriers in a world that increasingly requires technoliteracy. I've decided that one different thinker in my office who struggles with technology has dys-techia. We have built a number of accommodations around her and she now functions famously. In a world where we may soon only interact with learning through technology, a new (and probably misunderstood) subset of our population will face discrimination because of their technological limitations. If we plan well, though, this doesn't have to happen.

And if we speak up for *all* kids, not just the different thinkers, we won't have to repeat history. The lessons in this book are good for all kids. Accommodations? Good for everyone. Boosting self-esteem to facilitate resiliency so learning can actually happen? Essential for all students (but especially those who are struggling). My blueprint for an education revolution is simple. I promise you these lessons will help your kids follow in the steps of the many folks I have described in this book. Your kid will become Shena Vagliano or even Senator Bennet, if it's meant to be.

In this book, I have tried to put the lessons of Eye to Eye in your hands; I have no doubt your kids will be shining stars. If we don't speak up now, a population of different thinkers a generation in front of us will be at risk. And if we do, we can reshape the world for the better.

All it takes is one last step, starting with two words:

I am ...

Acknowledgments

Three days after my thirty-second birthday, I signed a contract with an amazing team at HarperCollins. I knew of other authors with dyslexia and ADHD who had written books, so it did not seem like I was making history. However, I wanted to be transparent about this process from day one. This book is a product of my community. I wrote this book with the help of coaches, editors, research assistants, and emotional support from a community of people at Eye to Eye and HarperCollins that is rare. All too often, we hold up individuals who have found success without knowing the whole story.

Here is the whole story.

To my mother, Vicki Flink: You are a truly talented educator and a loving mother. Thank you for all of your support throughout this journey and for allowing me to share our family's story so that others can find a smoother path. The students who are fortunate enough to have had you as their teacher benefit from your passion and your willingness to share equal parts heart and mind in every lesson. To my father, Barry Flink: You have shared with me your story with openness and generosity and allowed me to put a light on parts of our experiences for the world to see. Thank you for your love and support. Thank you to my uncle David Sotto, my grandfather Eli Sotto, and my whole extended family and in-laws for always being the shoulders for me to *learn* on. To my wife, Laura Flink: Thank you for being the most loving and compassionate partner a person could ever ask for. Wrapped in these pages are dreams you helped me unpack. If not for you, my life would be vacant of the power of the possible. Thanks for being with me on this journey. I love you.

Harold Koplewicz and Erica Jong: you both helped me find my story. To the whole Koplewicz family: you became my family when I moved to New York. Linda, Harold, Sam, Adam, and Josh: thank you for your generosity and commitment to service from which Eye to Eye grew. Harold and Erica: you also helped me find my incredible literary agent, Michael Carlisle. Thank you, Michael, for taking a risk on me. William Callahan: thanks for coming through when it really counted.

Lisa Cornelio: A player is only as good as he is coached. You were the best writing coach I could ever have wished for. More than that, your thought partnership and spirit support is without question why this project saw the light of day. The best is yet to come!

Henry Ferris and the whole HarperCollins gang: The day

we first met we created lightning in a bottle. To see that energy channeled into this project still amazes me. Thanks for taking a very raw manuscript and a very green writer and helping to create something lasting and special.

Marcus Soutra, Eye to Eye COO/Chief Intrapreneur/ friend: You moved to New York on faith that Eye to Eye could be huge. You see things in me and in Eye to Eye that I never believed possible, and without question your leadership and vision are what have made our work great. It is our friendship that has made it fun, too. Every word on these pages is a result of your hard work, loyalty to the mission, and dedication to excellence. I learn from you every day!

Vanessa Kirsch: As someone who strongly believes in the power of mentorship, you know I don't throw the word *mentor* around lightly. You are my mentor. Thank you for being a thought partner, ally, and friend from day one.

To the board, staff, and volunteer community of Eye to Eye: Our work is ongoing, but it is because of all of you that we have come this far. At the root of our daily commitment to the mission of Eye to Eye is the sharing of our stories, the owning of our experiences, and the willingness to operate with a sense of service to improve the lives of others with LD/ ADHD. You all are my role models and mentors.

Eye to Eye exists because of the visionary acts of generosity that remind me daily that change is possible because goodness lives within us all. I want to particularly thank the Eye to Eye funder community and donors—especially the Johnson Scholarship Foundation, the Oak Foundation, the Poses Family Foundation, the Emily Hall Tremaine Foundation, New Profit, Inc., and Prime Movers Hunt Alternative Fund. Wealth, wisdom, and web are the fabric of Eye to Eye, and as such what I once called an LD/ADHD "nudgement" is now a full-blown movement. Thank you for fueling our movement to make a world where one day all learners will be recognized.

At eighteen, I made two friendships that changed my life. David Hyman and Evan Michelson: thank you for your friendship and belief in me even before I believed in myself. Michael Zollinger: Few can say their childhood friends became life-long friends, but you are just that. Thank you for enriching my life from the day we met in middle school.

The stories from my childhood included in this book were stories not easily told. I chose to share them in the spirit of providing a window into an often invisible world of LD/ADHD. Many of these events happened a decade or two ago, and in no way am I attempting to defame individuals or institutions in this effort. I want to take a particular effort to acknowledge that both the Jewish day school and college prep school I attended in Atlanta are incredibly progressive institutions that have evolved tremendously in the past two decades and now do a wonderful job serving students with LD/ADHD. Thank you for allowing me to share stories of how we all learned together to create communities that are learning-oriented and willing to serve all students regardless of how they learn best.

Finally, I want to acknowledge that many of the stories in

this book come from others. Thus, in many ways, I did not write this book, but merely recounted it on behalf of them. There are also hundreds of stories that did not find their way to these pages. To those who volunteered their stories, but were not represented within this book: Know your stories mattered. Thank you for sharing them with me, and please continue to share them with others. This book is *our* book.

To that end, thank you, reader, for having the willingness to learn more, and I hope you find your own story in these pages. This is now your book, and I acknowledge your participation in continuing to write our collective story. While deeply grateful for the stories shared with me, I need this to be an evolving story. Please share your stories with me via eyetoeyenational.org and davidflink.com. I promise to read every story sent my way, collect them, and help wrap them in books that are yet to come. This is the beginning of a journey together. I acknowledge you.

Appendix: How to Be a Change Agent

While deeply grateful for the collective effort behind this book and the numerous stories and lessons that are shared within, I still need your help. I'd like you to share your stories with me—and the greater LD/ADHD community. I promise to read every submission. Ultimately, I'd like to include them in a future book on success in life after school/in the workplace and in future editions of this book. This is the beginning of our journey together.

Now I ask for one last promise. Don't let yours be an individual success. Make it one that can change education. Just follow the suggestions below.

Parents of People with LD/ADHD

1. Practice telling the story of how your child learns. Then help your child put words to this

experience (no matter how he or she chooses to tell it: art, music, poetry, writing, speeches, or just on the phone with a friend).

2. Tell someone that LD/ADHD is in your family. Then tell some more people.

3. Find allies among other parents who have children with LD/ADHD.

4. Find allies among people who don't know the LD/ADHD story and are willing to listen.

5. Stand up for your children at all costs, but especially around issues related to the LD/ADHD experience.

6. Don't lower the expectations for your children or any child. Keep the bar high, know they can all accomplish greatness, and be an example for your child.

7. Seek out role models with LD/ADHD for your children, both well known and unknown, but especially people they can speak with directly. Then become a partner for others.

8. If you see your child struggling in a way you once did, consider learning about your own experience and diving into your own history. You may have LD/ADHD and never been diagnosed. *You* might be your child's greatest LD/ADHD role model.

9. Learn how the disability rights movement helps define the rights of your child as someone with a learning disability. Learn about other civil rights movements too, so we don't have to redraw the map. The women's rights movement, the civil rights movement, and most recently, the gay rights movement are all excellent places to start.

10. Don't be afraid of accommodations for *all* children, which will help level the playing field. Seek them out early and when appropriate. Explain to your child that accommodations fix a broken education system, not a broken learner. Then help that practice become the norm. These things can be done at the grassroots level on school boards and at the federal level by speaking to your state representatives.

11. Help your school system and the children, teachers, and parents within understand that accommodations are not cheating. Then help all kids become comfortable asking for that help from others. Start practicing this at home or in a safe environment first.

12. Include your children in IEP and 504 meetings (if they are on IEP or 504 plans). Let them have a voice in these meetings as soon as possible.

13. Support fellow travelers with LD/ADHD and be a good listener; while there are common experiences across LD/ADHD, there is still diversity within this community. Get involved in social media (start by visiting the ETE Facebook page). Don't just read—share your thoughts and repeat them on your own social media pages. Follow up in the real world as well through community meet-up groups, and so on.

14. Know that today doesn't define tomorrow—it gets better!

15. Be conscious of the language you use; when you hear the words *stupid, lazy,* and so on, use your voice to be instructive.

16. Understand that we are part of a minority group and realize the powerful community that only grows with help.

17. Help your children understand that their LD/ADHD is *part* of who they are, but not the *sum* of who they are. The key is integration of identity, not compartmentalizing.

18. Help your child know his or her gifts— whether they derive from LD/ADHD or not.

19. Find ways for your children to use their gifts to support their weaknesses.

20. Seek out opportunities that help your children understand themselves better and become more well rounded.

21. Understand when your children are being defined based on rules that they did not set— for instance, *a good student learns while sit-*

ting still. Your child's worth is not defined by grades, and so on.

22. The keys to success can be boiled down to two components: know-how and agency. Help your children know how they learn best so they feel confident enough to ask for what they need. This story of success will create ripples!

23. What's next? Help us fill in the future ...

People with LD/ADHD

1. Practice telling the story of how you learn (no matter how you chose to tell it: art, music, poetry, writing, speeches, or just on the phone with a friend).

2. Tell someone. Then tell more people!

3. Seek out allies who have LD/ADHD.

4. Seek out allies who don't have LD/ADHD and are empathetic.

5. Seek out role models with LD/ADHD, both well known and unknown and especially people in your life whom you can speak with directly and share common experiences.

6. No matter what your age, tell people younger than you your story to support them on their journey—your experience is valuable!

7. Don't be afraid of accommodations.

8. Ask for accommodations and explain why you need them—use it as a teachable moment.

9. Support others with LD/ADHD and be good listeners; while people with LD/ADHD are a common people, we are still diverse.

10. Know that today doesn't define tomorrow—it gets better!

11. Be conscious of the language you use. If you hear *stupid, lazy,* and so on, know these words don't define you and you shouldn't use them to define others.

12. Understand your history—learn how the disability rights movement helps define the rights we have and where we are going.

13. Understand the concept of being a minority group, while still part of a powerful community that continues to grow.

14. Understand your LD/ADHD as *part* of who you are, but not the *sum* of who you are.

15. Know your gifts—whether they derive from your LD/ADHD or not.

16. Find ways to use your gifts to support your weaknesses.

17. Seek out opportunities that help you understand yourself better—become a more well-rounded person.

18. Understand when you define yourself based on your own rules and when others are defining you by rules that you did not set—your worth is not defined by your grades, what job you have, and so on.

19. Understand that LD/ADHD is not an excuse but an explanation for the need for accommodations.

20. What's next? Help us fill in the future . . . write us your thoughts at info@eyetoeyenational.org.

And . . . if you're a teacher and have students with LD/ADHD, strive to teach them in a variety of ways.

If you're an employer of people with LD/ADHD, strive to create work environments that allow them to accomplish tasks in a variety of ways.

If you don't fall into any of these groups, then talk to people with LD/ADHD to learn more about their life experiences.

Finally, go to the ETE Take Action Center to continue to develop this list and use dynamic tools to fuel our movement: http://eyetoeyenational.org/get_involved/gihome .html#raise.

Further Reading

Robert Brooks, Ph.D., and Sam Goldstein, Ph.D. *Raising Resilient Children: Fostering Strength, Hope, and Optimism in Your Child.* New York: Mc-Graw Hill, 2001.

Sam Chaltain, *Faces of Learning: 50 Powerful Stories of Defining Moments in Education.* San Francisco: Jossey-Bass, 2011.

Brock Eide, M.D., and Fernette Eide, M.D. *The Dyslexic Advantage: Unlocking the Hidden Potential of the Dyslexic Brain.* New York: Plume, 2011.

———. *The Mislabeled Child: How Understanding Your Child's Unique Learning Style Can Open the Door to Success.* New York: Hyperion, 2006.

Ben Foss. *The Dyslexia Empowerment Plan: A Blueprint for Renewing Your Child's Confidence and Love of Learning.* New York: Ballantine, 2013.

Malcolm Gladwell. *David and Goliath: Underdogs, Misfits, and the Art of Battling Giants.* Boston: Little, Brown, 2013.

Edward M. Hallowell, M.D., and John Ratey, M.D. *Driven to Distraction: Recognizing and Coping with Attention Deficit Disorder.* New York: Anchor Books, 2011.

Jane M. Healy, Ph.D. *Different Learners: Identifying, Preventing, and Treating Your Child's Learning Problems.* New York: Simon & Schuster, 2011.

Lederick R. Horne. *Rhyme Reason & Song* (audio CD).

Harold S. Koplewicz, M.D. *It's Nobody's Fault: New Hope and Help for Difficult Children and Their Parents.* New York: Three Rivers Press, 1996.

Rick Lavoie. *The Motivation Breakthrough: 6 Secrets to Turning On the Tuned-Out Child.* New York: Touchstone, 2007.

Mel Levine, M.D. *The Myth of Laziness: America's Top Learning Expert Shows How Kids—and Parents—Can Become More Productive.* New York: Simon & Schuster, 2003.

——. *A Mind at a Time: America's Top Learning Expert Shows How Every Child Can Succeed.* New York: Simon & Schuster, 2002.

Jonathan Mooney and David Cole. *Learning Outside the Lines: Two Ivy League Students with Learning Disabilities and ADHD Give You the Tools for Academic Success and Educational Revolution.* New York: Touchstone, 2000.

Kathleen G. Nadeau, Ph.D., Ellen B. Littman, Ph.D., and Patricia O. Quinn, M.D. *Understanding Girls with AD/HD*. Silver Spring, MD: Advantage Books, 1999.

Paul Orfalea. *Copy This!: Lessons from a Hyperactive Dyslexic Who Turned a Bright Idea into One of America's Best Companies*. New York: Workman, 2005.

Philip Schultz. *My Dyslexia*. New York: W.W. Norton & Co., 2011.

Sally Shaywitz, M.D. *Overcoming Dyslexia: A New and Complete Science-Based Program for Reading Problems at Any Level*. New York: Vintage Books, 2003.

Paul Tough. *How Children Succeed: Grit, Curiosity, and the Hidden Power of Character*. New York: Houghton Mifflin Harcourt, 2012.

Maryanne Wolf. *Proust and the Squid: The Story and Science of the Reading Brain*. New York: Harper Perennial, 2008.

Index

A

acceptance, of LD/ADHD,
274–277
accommodations, 145–169,
173–193. *See also* legal issues
accessibility to, 163–165
acquiring, 17, 99–104
advocating for, 177–182
compensatory mechanisms and,
182–184
defined, 145–146
empathy and, 266
environmental, 101, 128–131,
147–148, 165–167, 177–182,
223–224
evaluation for, 95–96 (*see also*
evaluation)
expectations and, 184–188
goals and, 188–193
importance of, 167–169, 173–177
medication as, 159–163
perception of, 162–163
range of, 146–149, 151–154
traditional *versus* asset-based,
149–151

visibility of, 154–158
acquired dyslexia, 40, 41
action plan, 83–113
acquiring accommodations,
99–104
advocating for child, 108–111
choosing evaluator, 89–93
documenting child's
development, 83–85
explaining evaluation to child,
96–99
preparing child for evaluation,
93–96
resources, 102, 105, 111–113
school selection and, 104–107
understanding legal rights,
85–89
Adderall. *See* medication
advocacy, 239–253
asking for accommodations,
177–182
benefits of, 239–243, 250–253
change and, 274–277, 287–293
communicating with school
personnel, 108–111

importance of, 18
making life choices and, 242
self-advocacy, 244–249
allies, 197–234
finding, 17, 201–205
listening by, 227–229
parents as, 197–201, 213–214,
222–234
peers as, 205–210
praise from, 214, 216–222
role models as, 210–216
alternative interventions, 112
American Psychological
Association, 59
Americans with Disabilities Act
(ADA)
defined, 87
understanding legal rights, 86
assessment. *See* evaluation
asset-based accommodations,
149–151
assistive technology
availability of, 102
feeling successful with, 251
importance of, 8, 168
technoliteracy and, 276
attention-deficit/hyperactivity
disorder (ADHD)
accepting, 274–277 (*see also*
identity)
ADD and, 43
defined, 39, 42, 43
gender and, 58–60
medication and, 8, 39, 159–163
as "other health impairment," 86
overcoming distractions,
123–126, 128–131
risks of, 59
Section 504 of the Rehabilitation
Act and, 103–104
symptoms of, 7

auditory processing disorder, 40, 42

B
Bach, Richard, 189–190
Bennet, Michael, 260–262
Boies, David, 48
book explosion (art project), 52–53
Bradley, Charles, 159
brain. *See also* learning style
fMRI (functional magnetic
resonance imaging), 44
intelligence, 26, 37–38
metacognition and, 118–120
thinking and learning style,
117–118
Branson, Richard, 190
Brown University, 11–12, 123–124,
151–154, 177–182, 184–188,
217–222, 247–249
bullying
by peers, 8–10, 72–77
by teachers, 154–158

C
Cass Business School, 190
Center for the Study of Learning
(Georgetown University), 45
Chaltain, Sam, 119, 120
child development, documenting,
83–85
Child Find Mandate, 87
Child Mind Institute, 25, 50, 67,
91, 157
Christensen, Clayton, 215
Civil Rights Project (UCLA),
215–216
Columbia University, 173–177,
249
combined ADHD, 42, 43
compensatory mechanisms,
182–184

confidence, importance of, 17, 27, 32
connection, with others, 268–274
correction, of effort, 122
Cruger, Matthew, 50, 91, 96

D
developmental dyslexia, 40
diet, importance of, 112
dis/Abilities Studies Program (Columbia University), 173–177
distractions, overcoming, 123–126, 128–131. *See also* attention-deficit/hyperactivity disorder (ADHD); environmental accommodations
documentation, of child's development, 83–85
dreaming, importance of, 126–128
Drive (Pink), 66–67
dyscalculia, 40, 41
dysgraphia, 40, 41
dyslexia. *See also* learning disabilities (LD)
"curing," 216–222
defined, 6–7, 40, 41
Dyslexic Advantage, The (Eide, Eide), 46–47
dyspraxia, 40

E
Eden, Guinevere, 45
Eide, Brock, 46–47, 48, 126
Eide, Fernette, 46–47, 126
Elementary and Secondary Education Act (ESEA), 259–262
empathy, 265–268
environmental accommodations
allies' help with, 223–224

importance of, 128–131, 147–148, 165–167, 177–182
least restrictive environment (LRE), 101
evaluation
avoiding, 27–33
choosing evaluators for, 89–93
explaining results to child, 96–99
importance of, 15–16
independent educational evaluation (IEE), 86
preparing child for, 93–96
privacy issues of, 90, 95
time needed for, 91–92
executive function, defined, 43
executive function disorder, 42
exercise, importance of, 112
Eye to Eye (ETE)
art-based curriculum of, 118–119, 135, 206–210
development of, 123–129, 133–137, 184–188
explanatory cards distributed by, 158
on facing learning disabilities, 24
founding of, 12
Independent Learning Experiment, 120
learning difference as focus of, 50
mentoring program of, 56–57, 154–156, 163–165, 205–216, 229–234, 250–253
national training conference, 191–193
nonprofit status of, 259–260
public speaking engagements, 257–258
on resilience, 77
staff of, 276
Strike Out Stigma, 263–265

Think Different Diplomats,
258–263
vision of, 12–14

F
failure
fear of, 126–128
overcoming, 123–126
F.A.T. City (videos), 60
fidgeting, 183–184, 231
financial issues
of finding resources, 32–33
private evaluation and, 90
Flink, David. *See also* Eye to Eye
(ETE)
accommodations used by,
128–131, 151–154
childhood of, 3–11, 62–65, 74–77,
197–205
college experience of, 11–12,
123–124, 151–154, 177–182,
184–188, 217–222, 247–249
DavidFlink.com, 129
ETE developed by, 11–14, 124–126
graduate school experience of,
173–177, 249, 265–266
public speaking by, 257–258
work experience of, 177–182
fMRI (functional magnetic
resonance imaging), 44
free appropriate public education
(FAPE)
defined, 87
public *versus* private schools, 105

G
Galloway School, 10, 76–77
gender
ADHD and, 58–60
learning disabilities (LD) and,
38–39

Georgetown University, 45
goals
exceeding expectations and,
188–193
learning style and, 126–128
Gosfield, Josh, 189
Greene, Maxine, 175–176

H
Hallowell, Ned, 159
Harvard University, 215
Hayes Street Elementary School,
51–55
heritability, of learning disabilities,
44–46
"high-stakes" (standardized) tests,
199–200, 259
Hobart and William Smith Colleges
(HWS), 163–165, 166, 230–234
homeschooling, 107
homework
helping child with, 32, 109–110
study habits for, 121
Horowitz, Sheldon, 37–38, 39
"hovering," by parents, 227–229

I
identity, 257–277
accepting LD/ADHD, 274–277
connecting with others, 268–274
empathy toward others and,
265–268
overcoming stigma of LD/
ADHD, 263–265
sharing stories about LD/
ADHD, 257–263, 290–293
impulsive ADHD, 42, 43
inattentive ADHD, 42, 43
independence, need for, 242
independent educational evaluation
(IEE), 86

Independent Learning Experiment
(Eye to Eye), 120
Individualized Education Program
(IEP), 16
advocacy by parents and,
108–111
developing, 96, 100–103
teachers' knowledge of, 147
Individuals with Disabilities
Education Act (IDEA)
defined, 87
impartial hearings required by
school, 104
least restrictive environment
(LRE) requirement, 101
public *versus* private schools,
104–106
"services plan," 105
special factors of, 102
understanding legal rights,
85–89
intelligence, 26, 37–38

J
Jet Blue, 190
Jonathan Livingston Seagull
(Bach), 189–190

K
kinesthetic learners, 150
Kinko's, 137–138
Kirsch, Vanessa, 25, 216
Koplewicz, Harold, 25, 28, 30, 38,
67, 69–70, 157
Kopp, Wendy, 136
Krause, Jennifer, 77–78, 88, 100

L
labeling, 49–50, 51–55
Lavoie, Rick, 60, 61
learning difference, defined, 50

learning disabilities (LD)
accepting, 274–277 (*see also*
identity)
bullying and, 8–10, 72–77, 154–158
causes of, 44–46
definitions, 37, 39–43
developing special talents and,
46–49, 56–57
gender and, 38–39
intelligence and, 37–38
labeling of, 49–50, 51–55
learning difference *versus,* 50
medication and, 39
motivation and, 58–60
resilience and, 77–79
self-esteem issues and, 60–61,
62–72
"learning hygiene," 167
"learning opportunities," 138
learning style, 117–140
advocacy and, 250–253
controlling environment
and, 128–131 (*see
also* environmental
accommodations)
developing skills for success, 122,
133–137
as individualized, 120–122
inspiration and, 126–128
kinesthetic learning, 150
learning as process and, 139–140
metacognition and, 118–120
for overcoming failure, 123–126
problem solving and, 137–139
risk taking and, 131–133
thinking differently and,
117–118, 140
traditional *versus* asset-
based accommodations
for, 149–151 (*see also*
accommodations)

understanding, 84
least restrictive environment
(LRE), 101
legal issues. *See also* Americans
with Disabilities Act (ADA);
Individualized Education
Program (IEP); Individuals
with Disabilities Education
Act (IDEA); Section 504 of
the Rehabilitation Act
private schools and, 104–106
school's obligations and, 33, 101
understanding legal rights,
85–89
life choices, independence and, 242
listening, importance of, 227–229
Logan, Julie, 190

M
medication
as accommodation, 159–163
for ADHD, 8
LDs and, 39
mentoring relationships. *See* Eye to
Eye (ETE)
metacognition, 118–120
mistakes, advantages of, 123–126
mixed dyslexia, 41
motivation, understanding LD/
ADHD and, 58–60, 108–109

N
National Center for Gender Issues
and ADHD, 59
National Center for Learning
Disabilities (NCLD)
on accommodations, 145–146
on documentation, 84–85
ETE partnership with, 259
on learning disabilities and
intelligence, 37–38, 39

Neeleman, David, 190
New Profit Inc., 25
New York Times, 189
No Child Left Behind, 259–262
nutrition, importance of, 112

O
Orfalea, Paul, 137–138
"other health impairments," 86
Otterbein, Piper, 78–79
overstimulation, problem of,
165–167

P
parents
as advocates, 239–243 (*see also*
advocacy)
as allies, 197–201, 213–214,
222–227, 229–234
as change agents, 285–290
child's development documented
by, 83–85
child's issues acknowledged
by, 5–6, 23–33 (*see also*
evaluation)
homework help and, 32, 109–110
listening by, 227–229
praise by, 61
Parent Training and Information
Centers (statewide), 106
peers
advocacy of, 244–247
as allies, 205–210
bullying by, 8–10, 72–77
phonological dyslexia, 41
Pink, Daniel, 66–67
praise
from allies, 214, 216–222
importance of, 61
prior written notice (PWN),
90–91

privacy
  accessibility to accommodations
    and, 163–165
  evaluation issues and, 90, 95
  visibility of accommodations
    and, 154–158
private evaluation, 90
private schools, legal issues of,
  104–106
problem solving, 137–139
progress, monitoring, 122

Q
Quinn, Patricia, 59

R
Rehabilitation Act. *See* Section 504
  of the Rehabilitation Act
remote evaluation services, 92
resilience, 77–79
resources, finding, 25, 32–33, 102,
  106, 111–113. *See also* schools
risk taking, 131–133
Ritalin. *See* medication
role models, 210–216. *See also*
  allies; Eye to Eye (ETE)

S
Schenck School, 6, 8–9, 64–65, 257
schools
  accommodation for school tests,
    146–147
  bullying and, 8–10, 72–77,
    154–158
  Child Find Mandate of, 87 (*see*
    also legal issues)
  compensating for dyslexia in,
    47–48
  finding allies in, 201–205
  impartial hearings required by,
    104

  perceived relevancy of, 126
  school as student's "job," 215
  selection of, 104–107
  self-esteem and, 64–66
  standardized testing by, 199–200,
    259
school tests. *See* testing
"Secret Ingredient for Success"
  (Sweeney, Gosfield), 189
Section 504 of the Rehabilitation
  Act
  defined, 103–104
  impartial hearings required by
    school, 104
  understanding legal rights, 16, 86
self-advocacy, 244–249, 290–293
self-awareness, 224–225
self-esteem
  importance of, 60–61
  learning style and, 127–128
  outside of school, 66–69
  overcoming shame for, 62–64,
    69–72
  in school, 64–66
self-injury, ADHD and, 59
semantic/dysnomia dyslexia, 41
sensory processing disorder, 40
"services plan," 105
shame, overcoming, 62–64, 69–72.
  See also self-esteem
Shaywitz, Sally, 149–150
sleep hygiene, 167
Soutra, Marcus, 161–162, 274
special education experts, 106
special factors, 102
special talents, developing, 46–49,
  56–57
specific learning disabilities
  (SLDs)
  defined, 42–43
  understanding legal rights, 85–89

standardized tests, 199–200, 259
stigma of LD/ADHD,
    overcoming, 263–265
stimulants, early use of, 159
Strike Out Stigma (ETE), 263–265
study habits, 121
success, developing skills for, 122,
    133–137, 250–253. *See also*
    advocacy; learning style
suicide risk, ADHD and, 59
"superhero project" (Eye to Eye),
    118–119
Super Parenting for ADHD
    (Hallowell), 159
support system. *see* allies
Sweeney, Camille, 189
symptoms, recognizing, 3–5, 15,
    27–31. *see also* evaluation

T
technology. *see* assistive
    technology
testing
  accommodation for school tests,
    146–147
  for learning disabilities (*see*
    evaluation)
  standardized tests, 199–200, 259
Think Different Diplomats (Eye to
    Eye), 258–263
traditional accommodations, 149–
    151. *See also* accommodations

U
Understanding Girls with AD/HD
    (Quinn), 59
University of California at Los
    Angeles (UCLA), 215–216
U.S. Senate, on LD/ADHD,
    259–262

V
Vagliano, Shena, 230–234, 263–264
video games, 68–69
Virgin Atlantic, 190
visual dyslexia, 41
visual processing disorder, 40, 42

W
workplace, accommodations in,
    177–182
writing centers, at universities, 220
Wyoming Department of
    Education, 77–78, 88, 100

Y
Yale Center for Creativity and
    Dyslexia, 149–150
Young Leaders Organizing
    Institute, 13
Your Learner Sketch (Chaltain),
    120

About the Author

In 1989, I was diagnosed with dyslexia and ADHD. I was nine years old. I grew up a member of the first generation of students to receive special education services and accommodations, but still I went through elementary, middle, and high school feeling helpless, hopeless, and lost. My parents and teachers assured me I'd be able to go to college one day, but I couldn't see how that was possible. Perhaps their message would have been more believable if it had come from a person with a learning disability who had gone to college and graduated.

I finally received the help I needed at an alternative high school. I began to excel academically and was even accepted to Brown University. However, I was marked by years of feeling inadequate. I was hungry for a community of people who'd had similar experiences in their early education. I also wanted to do something for younger students with learning disabilities.

In 1998, I cofounded Eye to Eye, a mentoring program for students with learning disabilities. The organization quickly grew from a small student-run initiative to a nonprofit with chapters across the country. As spokesperson for ETE, I have organized countless events for educators, parents, and students and lectured in hundreds of schools and universities. I established the Young Leaders Summit to train young people to lead grassroots campaigns and advocate for their rights as learners. In 2010, I was awarded a Prime Movers Fellowship, sponsored by the Hunt Alternatives Fund, which supports emerging and established social movement leaders who are developing innovative and inclusive approaches to social change. In 2013, Eye to Eye became part of the New Profit Portfolio, which also helped scale Teach for America.

I hold a bachelor's degree in education and psychology from Brown University and a master's degree in dis/Ability Studies in education from Columbia University.

I live with my wife, a physician, in New York City.